616.8527 ING   LAN

£30.50

DATE DUE			
1/4/16			

VULNERABILITY TO DEPRESSION

VULNERABILITY TO DEPRESSION

From Cognitive Neuroscience to Prevention and Treatment

RICK E. INGRAM
RUTH ANN ATCHLEY
ZINDEL V. SEGAL

THE GUILFORD PRESS
New York   London

© 2011 The Guilford Press
A Division of Guilford Publications, Inc.
72 Spring Street, New York, NY 10012
www.guilford.com

Printed in the United States of America

This book is printed on acid-free paper.

Last digit is print number: 9 8 7 6 5 4 3 2 1

Library of Congress Cataloging-in-Publication Data

Ingram, Rick E.
  Vulnerability to depression : from cognitive neuroscience to prevention
and treatment / Rick E. Ingram, Ruth Ann Atchley, and Zindel V. Segal.
      p. cm.
  Includes bibliographical references and index.
  ISBN 978-1-60918-255-7 (hardback)
  1. Depression, Mental—Risk factors.   2. Emotions and cognition.
3. Cognitive styles.   4. Depression, Mental—Treatment.   I. Atchley, Ruth Ann.
II. Segal, Zindel V., 1956–   III. Title.
  RC537.I544 2011
  616.85′27—dc22

                                                            2011011699

About the Authors

Rick E. Ingram, PhD, is Professor of Psychology at the University of Kansas. His research focuses on cognitive functioning in emotional disorders, with a particular emphasis on the cognitive features of individuals at risk for depression. This research examines the cognitive mechanisms of risk in adults, but also assesses processes linked to the possible developmental origins of cognitive risk. Dr. Ingram is the editor of the *International Encyclopedia of Depression*; coauthor (with Jeanne Miranda and Zindel V. Segal) of *Cognitive Vulnerability to Depression*; and currently editor of the journal *Cognitive Therapy and Research*. He is a recipient of the New Researcher Award from the Association for Advancement of Behavior Therapy (now the Association for Behavioral and Cognitive Therapies), the Distinguished Scientific Award for Early Career Contributions to Psychology from the American Psychological Association, and, most recently, the John C. Wright Graduate Mentor Award from the University of Kansas. He was also elected as a Division 12 Fellow of the American Psychological Association.

Ruth Ann Atchley, PhD, is Chair of the Department of Psychology and a member of the Cognitive and Clinical PhD Programs at the University of Kansas. Her research uniquely combines event-related-potential electrophysiological data with divided-visual-field research techniques to examine hemispheric differences in linguistic and other cognitive processes. With funding from a National Science Foundation grant, she investigated whether the left and right cerebral hemispheres contribute to the problems of language comprehension observed in readers with

a history of developmental language disorder. Related projects seek
to develop new measures of the perceptual and neurological processing abilities of children, older adults, and adults with early Alzheimer's
disease by assessing language abilities in tasks that require perceptual
processing, neurological processing, and off-line grammatical knowledge. Dr. Atchley has also spent the last 10 years investigating how neu-
rolinguistic processes contribute to the negative cognitive bias seen in
depressed individuals and those with chronic pain disorders. This work,
funded by the National Institute of Mental Health, examines behavioral
and electrophysiological markers that might help to predict depression
vulnerability and relapse. Most recently, she has extended this investigation of emotion and language to study more prosocial behaviors, such as
her work on generosity that is funded by the Templeton Foundation.

Zindel V. Segal, PhD, is the Cameron Wilson Chair in Depression Studies
and Head of the Mood and Anxiety Disorders Program in the Department of Psychiatry at the University of Toronto. He is also Head of
the Cognitive Behaviour Therapy Unit at the Centre for Addiction and
Mental Health and Professor in the Department of Psychiatry at the
University of Toronto. Dr. Segal has studied and published widely on
psychological treatments for depression for more than 25 years, especially the nature of psychological prophylaxis for this recurrent and dis-
abling disorder. He and his colleagues have pioneered the combined use
of mindfulness meditation and cognitive therapy as an effective relapse
prevention treatment. Dr. Segal's publications include *Mindfulness-
Based Cognitive Therapy for Depression* and *The Mindful Way through
Depression*, a patient guide that outlines this approach.

Preface

THE VULNERABLE PERSON

How can we describe the person who is vulnerable to depression? To start, our "typical" vulnerable person is most likely a woman. We can make this probability statement because we know that women are twice as likely as men to be diagnosed with depression. The risk for women to experience depression is thus considerably higher than for men. However, numerous other risk factors besides gender have been identified as well. For example, living in poverty, being divorced or separated, and smoking have been identified as risk factors, and we could have used these variables to refer to our vulnerable person, albeit not quite as easily. So, for the time being, in describing vulnerability, it makes sense to think of our vulnerable person as a woman.

Before going further, however, it is important to point out that a risk factor, gender in this case, is significant but not informative about vulnerability because it does not tell us about the processes or mechanisms that bring about depression. Being female means she has a greater chance of becoming depressed, but it does not tell us why this is the case. Later in this book we will expand on the differences between risk and vulnerability, but, in short, risk tells us about the probability of becoming depressed, whereas vulnerability tells us about the processes involved in becoming depressed.

So, how can we describe our vulnerable woman, and, more specifically, what do we know about her cognitive and neurological processes that make her vulnerable? And how did these processes come about? We paint some aspects of this picture here with very broad strokes and fill in the details in the various chapters of this book. We start the picture with cognitive processes.

COGNITIVE VULNERABILITY

There is a considerable body of evidence to show that depressed people think in a negatively biased way, particularly in reference to themselves. The most concise description of this kind of thinking is provided by Aaron Beck in his negative cognitive triad: depressed people think in unrealistically negative terms about themselves, their world, and the future.

Does our currently nondepressed but vulnerable person also evidence the negative cognitive triad? She does not if things are generally going fine, but a sufficiently negative life event, or a series of events, can trigger the negative cognitive triad. This negative thinking may form the core of a rumination process, or, as it was described a number of years ago, a cognitive recycling process whereby negative thoughts are recycled throughout conscious and subconscious thinking. Benign events are then interpreted as negative, and genuinely negative events are interpreted as even more negative than they really are.

The preoccupation with negative thinking and the preponderance of negative thoughts make problem solving difficult. In the face of these thinking biases, she may receive social support, but the continuing negativity makes it difficult to maintain this support. People want to help, but their support proves ineffective because it is undermined by the negative biases, which eventually drive people to distance themselves. This distancing creates a cycle in which support seeking intensifies, which drives support further away, further intensifying support seeking. These cognitive and social/interpersonal processes, instigated by her negative cognitive self-schema, create a spiral into a depressed state.

What is the origin of schemas like hers? The evidence suggests that they are most likely created from adverse events in childhood. The possible originating events are myriad and not easily mapped directly to later depression, but disruptions in the normal attachment process and ruptured bonding between parents and their children seem to play a role. Some of these experiences may involve abuse, yet not all depressed women were abused, and not all abused women eventually become depressed. Such abuse is certainly virulent, but may be placed in the broader context of attachment and bonding disruptions that create the fertile conditions for the creation of the negative cognitive schema.

VULNERABILITY FROM A NEUROSCIENCE PERSPECTIVE

In this book, cognitive vulnerability refers to mental processes such as attention (at least at a conscious level), memory, beliefs, thinking, reasoning, and decision making. As we just noted, and as we will discuss in detail later, in our vulnerable woman these mental processes coalesce around negatively biased thinking. What can cognitive neuroscience data show us about our vulnerable person? Although numerous neuroanatomical structures and connections may be involved in vulnerability, the research has shown us some that appear to be particularly important. Of key relevance appear to be the cingulate gyrus, prefrontal cortex, and, in the limbic system, the amygdala and hippocampus. Thus, our vulnerable person may have a prefrontal cortex (perhaps only on the left side) and cingulate gyrus that are chronically underactivated, and a limbic system that is hyperactivated. Or relative to nonvulnerable people, she may demonstrate, respectively, a tendency toward frontal underactivation and limbic hyperactivation in response to negative events, such as criticism. In sum, the cognitive neuroscience data suggest that our vulnerable woman shows less neocortical activity in some key brain regions, and a tendency toward greater responsiveness in other brain regions, particularly in subcortical structures that are part of the critical limbic system.

As we proceed through the chapters in this book, we will elaborate on these ideas and point to the evidence that supports them. We will also integrate, where possible, the cognitive and neurocognitive perspectives on vulnerability, and additionally discuss the treatment options available for our vulnerable person. To do so, we start in Chapter 1 with an overview of the public problem that is depression by defining the disorder and describing its diagnosis, its epidemiology, and its correlates and features. In Chapter 2 we describe the idea of vulnerability itself and also discuss its definition and its origins, as well as its differentiation from risk. In Chapter 3 we describe the basic ideas that underlie cognitive–clinical and cognitive neuroscience approaches to understanding behavior; then, in Chapter 4 we examine the methodological strategies that are important to understanding vulnerability from the standpoint of these approaches. In Chapter 5 we examine the theory and data that inform our understanding of the cognitive factors operating in vulnerability, while in Chapter 6 we address the cognitive neuroscience data on vulnerability. In Chapter 7 we examine the overlap between these perspectives and their points of departure. In Chapter 8 we discuss the clinical translation of cognitive and neuroscience views of vulnerability, and, based on these views, underscore patient factors that may contribute to the prevention of depression. In Chapter 9 we focus on the clinical outcomes for treatments that aim to teach patients how to address depression risk factors. Finally, in Chapter 10 we revisit our vulnerable person and reexamine the vulnerability from the perspectives and data we examined in the preceding chapters. The perspectives on depression we develop in this book, based on the notions of vulnerability and cognition, provide key insights to the disorder, where is comes from, how it debilitates people, and how we can work to prevent and treat it.

Contents

1

Depression

An Overview of a Public Health Problem

Prior to examining risk for depression, we examine the disorder itself. Just what is depression, and how is it conceptualized within current diagnostic systems? In this chapter we explore those questions, including the subtypes and diverse features of depression, discuss the epidemiology of depression, and examine the correlates and features of depression—including gender differences in the prevalence of the disorder, as well as the complex impact of cultural forces in depression. We discuss morbidity and comorbidity as well.

THE DEPRESSION CONSTRUCT

How depression is conceptualized has important implications for how vulnerability is understood. At its simplest level, the definition of a depression also defines how we understand vulnerability. For example, to what is the individual vulnerable: a symptom, a psychological syndrome, a physical disease, or some other configuration of depressive symptoms? How depression is defined also has implications for understanding at what point high-risk people transition from vulnerability to depression to the depressed state itself. To the extent that depression is defined in a categorical fashion, that point comes when individuals meet five out of a possible nine symptoms as specified by the *Diagnostic and Statistical Manual of Mental Disorders* (4th ed., text rev. [DSM-IV-TR; American

Psychiatric Association, 2000]). However, a view of vulnerability that adheres to a dimensional approach might conceptualize transition to disorder at a different point.

To date, most if not all vulnerability theories and data are based on a categorical view of depression, but if this definition of depression is revised at some point, then vulnerability ideas may require similar revision. Likewise, if "depression" is in fact a term for a causally heterogeneous set of conditions that eventuate in various depressive symptoms, vulnerability theory and research would potentially need to consider a set of vulnerability theories and data to match different causal pathways. Vulnerability theory and research has not yet grappled with these possibilities and issues, but may need to do so in the future if our understanding of risk is to be accurate. As such, we believe that any discussion of vulnerability to depression must also include an examination of the issues and perspectives that inform how we define depression, as well as an examination of some the strengths and limitations of various definitions.

Defining Depression

In North America, the definition, description, and diagnostic criteria for depression are currently governed by the DSM-IV-TR (American Psychiatric Association, 2000). This edition will soon be supplanted by the fifth edition of the DSM, but because it seems unlikely that DSM-5 will reflect major changes in depression description and diagnostic criteria, we proceed with our discussion based on the information provided by DSM-IV-TR. Before doing so, however, a number of caveats are in order.

Depression can be thought of in a variety of ways. For instance, Nurcombe (1992) argued that "depression" can describe a mood state, a symptom or sign, a dynamic constellation of conscious or unconscious ideas, a syndrome consisting of a constellation of symptoms, a disorder that allows for the identification of a group of individuals, or a disease that is associated with biochemical or structural abnormalities. Likewise, Kendall, Hollon, Beck, Hammen, and Ingram (1987) noted different levels of reference to which depression can refer; the term depression

> has several levels of reference: symptom, syndrome, nosological disorder (Beck, 1967; Lehmann, 1959). Depression itself can be a symptom—for example, being sad. As a syndrome, depression is a

constellation of signs and symptoms that cluster together (e.g., sad-ness, negative self-concept, sleep and appetite disturbances). The syn-drome of depression is itself a psychological dysfunction but can also be present, in secondary ways, in other diagnosed disorders. Finally, for depression to be a nosological category, careful diagnostic proce-dures are required during which other potential diagnostic categories are excluded. (p. 290)

An idea implicit in this description is that the most appropriate way to understand depression is to view it as one category among different categories of psychological disorders, an approach that is adhered to by DSM-IV-TR and its recent predecessors.

While the taxonomic systems that typically underlie scientific clas-sification divide variables into categories, descriptions of psychological disorders can represent an exception. That is, psychological disorders can be conceptualized as categories or as dimensions. Dimensional approaches are inherently quantitative in nature and suggest that clinical depression is an extension of normal sadness and mild depressive states, albeit an extreme extension. On the other hand, categorical approaches are defined by qualitative distinctions, and thus, while they share an emotion, clinical depression is seen as a fundamentally different psy-chological state than normal sadness and mild depression. Categorical distinctions also assume that different disorders represent different con-ditions with relatively discrete boundaries between them.

As noted, DSM-IV-TR employs a categorical approach to describing disorders, which are depicted as discrete nosological entities that occur independently of other nosological entities. DSM-IV-TR, of course, pro-vides the caveat that disorders are not necessarily true categorical vari-ables:

DSM-IV is a categorical classification that divides mental disorders into types based on criteria sets with defining features. ... There is no assumption that each category of mental disorder is a completely discrete entity with absolute boundaries dividing it from other mental disorders or from no mental disorder. There is also no assumption that all individuals described as having the same mental disorder are alike in all important ways. (American Psychiatric Association, 2000, p. xxxi).

Such a qualification in the preface of DSM-IV-TR is important and nec-essary, but the manual nevertheless promulgates a categorical system for understanding clinically meaningful psychological distress. Not surprisingly, this categorical system has been widely accepted by psychiatrists and psychologists as well as by institutions such as the National Institutes of Health and insurance companies that offer some reimbursement for the treatment of disorders. No one reads prefaces.

Several researchers have, however, advocated for a dimensional approach to depression, as well as for other disorders (e.g., Widiger & Samuel, 2005). Others have argued for an approach that incorporates both categorical and dimensional approaches (e.g., Kessler, 2002; Kessler & Wang, 2009). Klein (2008) suggested that DSM-5 presents an opportunity to reconsider how depression is conceptualized and suggests that depression could be dimensionally classified according to severity and chronicity. There are a number of advantages to adopting a dimensional approach, or at least an approach that incorporates dimensional aspects. For example, dimensional approaches offer a considerable degree of information beyond what is available in a categorical approach that describes an individual as either depressed or not depressed. Beyond the clinical utility of such information, research would see several advantages such as the greater statistical power that comes with a dimensional as opposed to a dichotomous framework. Thus, there has been considerable interest in developing a dimensional model to replace the categorical approach used by the DSM, but whether DSM-5 will adopt such a view is currently unknown.

Of course, whether the underlying structure of depression is dimensional or categorical is unknown. Some research has suggested the dimensionality of the disorder, at least with mild or subclinical levels of the disorder on one end of the dimension and clinical depression on the other end (e.g., Solomon, Haaga, & Arnow, 2001). Other research has supported a categorical approach (Solomon, Ruscio, Seeley, & Lewinsohn, 2006). It is also possible that depression may have both dimensional and categorical features. Hence, depression might be classified as a dimensional variable that once one passes a threshold on severity, for example, is classified as a disorder. Such a system might well capture the dimensional properties of the disorder while at the same making use of the advantages of a categorical approach (Kessler, 2002).

Advantages of Categorical Approaches

Despite criticisms of categorical approaches, a categorical framework to the conceptualization of psychological disorders does have a number of advantages. Reflecting the fact that the ability to categorize underlies all language and communication, categorical terms for psychological conditions are easily understood and thus facilitate communication between and among professionals and laypeople. Moreover, categorical perspectives simplify the conceptualization of psychopathology, at least relative to dimensional approaches, and thus can expedite clinical decision-making processes (Trull, Widiger, & Guthrie, 1990).

The categorical approach that has worked well in medicine is thus an explicitly disease- or illness-based approach. By extension, at least for some investigators, psychological disorders represent another disease category. Hence, a psychological disorder "is a medical disorder whose manifestations are primarily signs or symptoms of a psychological (behavioral) nature" (Spitzer & Endicott, 1978, p. 18). Depression is therefore another category of medical disorder or illness, a view that if correct strongly argues for the use of discrete categories.

Limits of Categorical Approaches

Syndromes versus Symptoms

Categorical approaches to psychological disorders such as that espoused by DSM-IV-TR are not without limitations. Irrespective of whether disorders like depression reflect true categories, or are better served by a dimensional approach, researchers have long pointed out the limitations of relying solely on a categorical approach to define and then study psychopathology. Persons (1986), for example, notes that theories are often explicitly tied to psychological phenomena and if research is limited only to diagnostic categories, important psychological phenomena may be ignored or missed. Consider suicidality, a problem that afflicts depression but is also associated with other problems (e.g., anxiety and physical illness). If suicide is only studied within the diagnostic category of depression, then important aspects of this phenomenon may be missed. Conversely, focusing on suicidality irrespective of diagnostic category allows for the study of individuals who share this problem, and are thus alike in important ways. This approach may thus be better able to uncover mechanisms that underlie disordered behavior and can therefore facilitate theoretical development in ways that studying a diagnostic category cannot. Moreover, the diagnostic category approach implicitly assumes that individuals with the same diagnosis are identical, an assumption that we turn to now.

Uniformity Assumptions

DSM-IV-TR explicitly cautions that people with depression are not alike in all important ways. Yet a categorical approach works strongly against this caveat. For instance, in the course of most research, the assumption that depression is a uniform disorder is implicitly made by recruiting research participants who meet diagnostic criteria for depression. Results are typically reported for the depressed group without acknowledgment of the heterogeneous group of symptoms represented within the group.

The assumption of uniformity, either explicitly or implicitly, is thus clearly incorrect. Consider that DSM-IV-TR lists nine symptoms, five of which are necessary for a diagnosis. However, this means that two people with the identical diagnosis of depression might share only one symptom in common. Although both of these people are "depressed," they are also different in potentially important ways, differences that may outweigh their similarities. Likewise, an individual who has experienced five symptoms for 14 days is likely quite different from the person who has experienced all nine symptoms for 6 months, but both are "simply" depressed. There are also differences within the symptoms themselves. For example, the symptom of sleep disturbance can be reflected in initial insomnia, middle insomnia, or terminal insomnia. Similarly, appetite change can refer to loses or gains in appetite. Hence, even when two depressed individuals share a symptom, this symptom can reflect polar opposites in these individuals.

Differences within the subjective quality or experience of symptoms can also occur. For example, one person may have a very different subjective experience of sadness than does another, yet both are considered identical when it comes to this symptom. In a similar fashion, differences in the temporal relationship between symptoms may also occur; some symptoms may arise or be severe during some points within the disorder, while other symptoms may occur or be severe at other points. The categorical approach incorporated into DSM-IV-TR cannot distinguish such differences.

In a categorical approach, the individual who does not meet criteria for a disorder does not have a disorder. Hence, a corollary aspect of the uniformity assumption is that the depressed individual is always different in important ways from the "nondepressed" person. This assumption is, however, unfounded. To illustrate, Wells et al. (1989) found that medical patients with depressive symptoms that did not reach criteria for depression nevertheless experienced as much disability as did those who met criteria for major depression. Likewise, Klein (2008) has noted that dysthymia is viewed as a milder disorder, but in many cases has been empirically shown to reflect more impairment than major depression.

Subtypes, Etiologies, Diverse Features, and the Reification of Depression

Most, if not the majority, of explicit discussions about the nature of depression note the heterogeneity of depression, that what is referred to as "depression" is not a uniform disorder but instead reflects a group of depressions. Some of the expression of this heterogeneity can be seen in discussions of subtypes of depression. For example, common divisions of depression in the past have seen discussion of neurotic versus psychotic depression, or melancholic versus psychological depression, or endogenous versus reactive depression. Some subtypes have been proposed on theoretical grounds as a way to bring clarity to research findings, such as Abramson and Alloy's (1990) proposal for a cognitive subtype of depression. Other subtypes have been officially incorporated into diagnostic systems, along with various specifiers. Thus, DSM-IV-TR lists not only major depressive disorder but also dysthymia. But major depressive disorder can be further differentiated as having postpartum features, atypical features, seasonal features, psychotic features, and melancholic features.

Another distinction that can be made is between depression and bereavement, a state that has all the features of depression, but that is not considered depression. We note parenthetically that Beckham, Leber, and Youll (1995) point out an interesting irony that results from diagnostically differentiating bereavement and depression. Even though the underlying processes may be identical, they observe that the woman who experiences significant depressive symptoms following the death of her husband will not be considered to have a disorder, yet the woman who experiences precisely the same symptoms after her husband leaves her will qualify for a depression diagnosis.

Considerations of heterogeneity and subtypes highlight the fact that depression is a construct. It is a group of symptoms, which are themselves constructs, that mental health professionals attempt to fit together in some meaningful way. In so doing, however, it can be argued that we have reified the construct. That is, by developing formal diagnostic criteria for major depressive disorder, and by employing a nosological/categorical/disease-based conceptualization, mental health researchers and clinicians have imbued depression with a reality that is separate from a psychological construct.

In observing the reification of the depression construct, we do not mean to suggest that criteria be discarded, or even that a categorical way of communicating about psychological states be eliminated. Owing to the prevalence of depressive states (i.e., co-occurring symptom constellations) and their associated impairment, the depression construct is arguably the most important construct in psychology and psychiatry. Moreover, assessing the construct in as reliable, valid, and objective a manner as is possible is crucial. Rather, we mean to suggest that is important that researchers be cognizant of the constructed nature of the disorder and how it is conceptually and empirically treated. It appears, however, that official criteria and the reliance on these criteria in judging the quality of grant proposals and manuscript submissions, and the validity of health insurance claims, tends to discourage consideration of the meaning of the construct. DSM criteria reflect an important and useful operational definition of an idea that has taken on its own certain truth.

Having noted issues with how depression is conceptualized and reified, we turn now to a description of depression that is, predictably, based on DSM criteria. As we have noted, categorical approaches are necessary for communalization, and our task of discussing vulnerability is eased considerably by the availability of such categories. But in so doing, we attempt to remain aware of the constructed nature of depression, and even as we rely on DSM-IV-TR, we note explicitly that this is but one of potentially many different operational definitions of the depression idea.

DEFINITION AND DESCRIPTION OF DEPRESSION

Symptoms

There are two cardinal symptoms of depression; that is, at least one or the other must be present before a diagnosis can be made. The first and most self-evident is depressed mood that, according to diagnostic criteria, must be present most of the day for at least 2 weeks. The second, and less self-evident, cardinal symptom is a loss of interest or pleasure in nearly all activities (i.e., anhedonia). Of course, these cardinal symptoms are not mutually exclusive and can co-occur in the depressed individual.

It should be noted, however, that anhedonia is infrequent compared to other depressive symptoms, and is much less frequent than depressed mood (see Weissman, Bruce, Leaf, Flirio, & Holzer, 1991).

There are a myriad of possible symptoms of depression that could be recognized, but beyond these two cardinal symptoms, DSM-IV-TR only "officially recognizes" seven other symptoms, making for a total of nine possible symptoms. In addition to at least one of the cardinal symptoms being present, a diagnosis of depression requires at least four of the nine symptoms. Of course, beyond the five-symptom minimum threshold, many cases of depressive disorder are associated with all nine symptoms, although it is important to recognize that they may not all be experienced with equal severity or during the same time-frame. These additional symptoms include significant weight gain or weight loss, insomnia or hypersomnia, psychomotor agitation or retardation, fatigue or loss of energy, feelings of worthlessness or excessive guilt, a diminished ability to think or concentrate, and recurrent thoughts of death or suicidal ideation, a suicide plan, or suicide attempts.

Age of Onset

When does depression occur? The modal age of onset of a depressive episode is in early adulthood. Thus, individuals in their late teens and early to mid-20s can be considered to be at the highest risk. For example, the National Institute of Mental Health Epidemiologic Catchment Area (ECA) study showed that 20% of cases met criteria for diagnosis for the first time before the age of 25 years, and 50% before age 39 (Dryman & Eaton, 1991). However, depression can occur at any age—even in early and middle childhood, although this is uncommon. Depression rates begin to increase substantially in adolescence (Garber, Gallerani, & Frankel, 2009). Interestingly, though irritability is not a symptom of adult depression, depressed children and adolescents display increased irritability as a core symptom (Kessler & Wang, 2009).

Depression in the elderly is less common than depression in younger individuals (see Kessler et al., 2010). Some evidence suggests that depression in the elderly and in children may be of an atypical, and more difficult-to-treat, nature than the depression seen in late adolescence and early adulthood. Early onset in childhood also suggests a poor prognosis for lifetime functioning (Costello, 2009). Depression can be chronic and frequently recurring (Boland & Keller, 2009), and early onset may thus reflect an increased risk of chronicity (Costello, 2009).

DEPRESSION EPIDEMIOLGY

Epidemiology is the study of the incidence of a disorder along with variables associated with its course and prognosis. Most of the existing epidemiological research in depression is descriptive or analytic in nature.

Prevalence Rates

Epidemiological data assess the incidence of a disorder in several ways. *Point prevalence rates* assess the incidence of a disorder at a particular point in time and is obtained in epidemiological surveys by assessing the number of individuals who meet criteria for depression at the time of the survey. As such, point prevalence rates can be thought of as a snapshot of the incidence of the number of depressed people at a given time. Not all epidemiological studies report point prevalence rates, however. A close cousin of point prevalence is the *1-month prevalence rate*, the rate at which people experience a depressive episode in the preceding month.

Twelve-month prevalence rates reflect the number of individuals who reported having experienced a depressive episode at some point during the preceding year, and thus reflect a broader examination of the incidence of depression. *Lifetime prevalence data* are typically gathered retrospectively and aim to estimate the percentages of individuals who have or will experience depression over the course of their lifetimes.

Several epidemiological surveys have gathered data about the prevalence rates of depression. The first was the National Institute of Mental Health ECA study, which interviewed over 20,000 adults in five states (Eaton & Kessler, 1985; Eaton et al., 1984; Regier et al., 1988). The ECA used the Diagnostic Interview Schedule (Robins, Helzer, Croughan, & Ratcliff, 1981) to diagnose dysthymia and major depression (among other disorders) according to the criteria of DSM-III. The data from all sites were merged and standardized to the 1980 U.S. population to provide an estimate of national prevalence rates (Regier et al., 1988).

A decade later, between 1990 and 1992, the National Comorbidity Survey (NCS; Kessler et al., 1994) was conducted using a modified version of the World Health Organization's (WHO) Composite International Diagnostic Interview (CIDI) to diagnose disorders, including depression, according to the DSM-III criteria. As such, the NCS was the first study to survey a representative national sample in the United States. Most recently, the National Comorbidity Survey—Replication, which again included depression (NCS-R; Kessler et al., 2003), was conducted. Like the original NCS, the replication surveyed a large number of individuals, approximately 9,000 respondents over the age of 18 in the 48 contiguous states. The NCS-R, however, used the criteria promulgated in DSM-IV, and assessed these criteria with an extended form of the CIDI (Kessler et al., 2003). The change to DSM-IV is important because it is not only the most current diagnostic system, but it also emphasizes clinical significance in diagnosis. Indeed, some have suggested that depression prevalence rates reported in the ECA and NCS were unrealistically high because many clinically questionable cases were diagnosed.

Point Prevalence Rates

Point prevalence rate data have not been reported by the ECA, NCS, or NCS-R. However, some data are available via the WHO's International Consortium on Psychiatric Epidemiology (ICPE), an endeavor that seeks to consolidate data from international epidemiological surveys. In various samples reported by the ICPE, point prevalence rates are between 2 and 4% for various samples of adults (Kessler & Wang, 2009).

One-Month Prevalence Rates

Of the three major surveys in the United States, only the ECA study reports 1-month prevalence rates. In particular, the ECA study found that approximately 2.2% of the sample experienced a major depressive episode over a 1-month period. As we noted, 1-month prevalence rates are closely related to point prevalence rates, suggesting that a somewhat higher than 2% prevalence rate may represent a reasonably accurate snapshot of current depression rates.

Twelve-Month Prevalence Rates

Twelve-month prevalence rates reported by the ECA study are the lowest of all the surveys, with findings indicating a rate of 2.7%. The NCS, on the other hand, found a 12-month prevalence rate almost twice as high, at 4.9%. The rate was higher still in the NCS-R findings, with a rate of 6.6%.

Lifetime Prevalence Rates

Lifetime prevalence rates for major depressive disorder are again the lowest in the ECA study, with a reported rate of 2.7%. The NCS rate in adults, defined as over 15, was substantially higher, with a reported rate of 15.8%. The NCS-R data are a little higher, but roughly in line with the NCS, with a reported rate of 16.6%.

As can be seen, the rates vary substantially, owing probably to different assessment methods, different samples, and different diagnostic criteria. The best available science seems to be evidenced by the NCS-R, lending weight to the various estimates reported by this survey, although rates will of course vary depending on how depression is operationally defined. Nevertheless, even the lowest rates reported in these large-scale studies are cause for concern. A point and 1-month prevalence rate in excess of 2–4% may not sound serious at first glance, but by analogy such a rate of the H1N1 (swine) flu would be enough to declare a worldwide pandemic.

Course of Depression

To examine the course of depression, we briefly note some of the key terms that define course. Specifically, *onset* refers to the transition from a nonsymptomatic, or subsymptomatic, state to one that meets criteria for depression. Meeting these criteria defines an episode of depression. The *maintenance* of the disorder reflects the persistence of it over some period of time. *Remission* can be seen as partial, where the individual no longer meets criteria for depression, but some symptoms are still evident. *Full remission*, on the other hand, has no or only few symptoms. *Recovery* also refers to a lack of symptoms, but is defined as being symptom-free (or symptom-minimal) over a longer period of time. Remission implies that, although the individual is free of clinically significant symptoms, his or her disorder may still be present. Recovery, however, assumes that the disorder is no longer present.

The assumption in remission that the underlying disorder may still be present not only has significant consequences for understanding the nature of the depression, but may also convey important information about the adequacy of treatment interventions. An important dimension in differentiating remission from recovery is the duration of the symptom-free period, yet there is no consensus about that dimension. Recently, however, Rush et al. (2006) have suggested guidelines that show promise for forming the basis of some consensus. In particular, they have suggested that remission be defined as a period of 3 consecutive weeks wherein individuals have no more than minimal symptoms, and do not meet diagnostic criteria; hence neither sad mood nor anhendonia is present, nor are more than three of the remaining DSM-IV-TR-described symptoms present.

Many cases of depression appear to be time-limited, although estimates vary as to the "natural" time course of depression in these cases. For instance, some data suggest that untreated depression can last between 6 months and 1 year (Dorzab, Baker, Winokur, & Cadoret, 1971; Keller, Shapiro, Lavori, & Wolfe, 1982), and others imply a time range of between 4 and 9 months (Depression Guideline Panel, 1993). Other data indicate that untreated depressed individuals recover, on average, in about 3 months. The range is obviously quite wide, but suggests that if an individual will naturally recover, it will not be a matter of a few days, but will also not be longer than a year. Although this range defines most cases of recovery, some cases of untreated major depression can remain symptomatic for up to 2 years. These differences in time to natural recovery may have potentially important implications for understanding vulnerability. For example, does depression with a long time to recovery carry with it a greater vulnerability to recurrence relative to a shorter time to recovery?

Much of the information we have on the course of depression is "confounded" because most data examine remission and recovery rates in treated samples; we do not have a wealth of evidence on the course of depression in untreated persons. Looking at treated samples, though, different studies report a range of results—from a high of over 70% of patients recovering within 1 year (Ormel et al., 1993) to a low of 35% (Simon et al., 2004).[1] Most studies find recovery happens in some period between these estimates, and all of them show that the majority of patients recover with treatment (see Boland & Keller, 2009). However, a very small percentage of patients, up to 10% in some research, do not recover even with treatment.

In sum, many patients recover or enter remission without treatment, although it may take up to a year in some cases, and when treated the majority of patients recover. However, recovery and remission rates tell us only some of the story of the course of depression because many

[1]It should be noted that Simon et al. used a very conservative definition of recovery, specifically the disappearance of *all* symptoms.

patients experience relapse or recurrence. For example, Keller et al. (1983) reported that 22% of remitted patients relapsed within a year. High rates of recurrence have been found in several studies, and the difference among findings may be a function to some degree of the length of follow-up time; longer periods provide a greater "opportunity" for recurrence, and indeed more recurrence is seen the longer we look out from the index episode. Hence, data from the Collaborative Depression Study (Katz, Secunda, Hirschfeld, & Koslow, 1979) show that recurrence rates within 2 years are as high as 40%, and are 87% after 15 years (Boland & Kessler, 2009). Moreover, Boland and Kessler (2009) note that after 20 years in their study, only 9% of the original sample had not relapsed.

Clearly, relapses and recurrences are common even after treatment. A number of variables have been found to be associated with relapse and recurrence, among them early or late onset, number of previous episodes, and poverty. The nature of treatment received may also play an important role. In large studies assessing relapse and recurrence, treatment is often monitored but not controlled or administered as an independent variable (Boland & Keller, 2009). These studies thus represent a hodgepodge of treatments with varying efficacies and possible prophylactic effects. There are data, however, to suggest that individuals treated with cognitive therapy, or a combination of cognitive therapy and psychopharmacology, are considerably less likely to experience relapse or recurrence than is the norm (Hollon, Stewart, & Strunk, 2006), possibly due to that intervention's specific efforts to modify underlying risk processes in the form of cognitive schemas (see Garret, Ingram, Rand, & Sawalani, 2007).

CORRELATES AND FEATURES OF DEPRESSION

Although epidemiological surveys evidence the extent of depression, they do not tell the whole story because depression is associated with a number of variables.

Gender Differences

Compared to men, women are at a much higher risk for depression. Although female-to-male ratios differ somewhat across studies, the average ratio is close to 2:1 (Nolen-Hoeksema, 1987; Weissman & Klerman,

1977, 1985; Weissman, Leaf, Holzer, Meyers, & Tischler, 1984). Prevalence rates for depression vary across different countries, but this gender difference remains (Nolen-Hoeksema & Hilt, 2009). Moreover, within the United States, this difference holds generally for African American, Latina, and Caucasian women and tends to persist even when income, education, and occupation are controlled (Radloff, 1975; Williams, Teasdale, Segal, & Kabat-Zinn, 2007).

As with most findings, this difference was found in the NCS, with women having a lifetime prevalence of 21.3% and men a lifetime prevalence of 12.7%. Further analysis of these data (Kessler, McGonagle, Swartz, Blazer, & Nelson, 1993), as well as data from the NCS-R (Kessler et al., 2003), reveal some interesting differences, and similarities, across genders. For example, women are much more likely than men to develop a first episode of depression, but men and women develop first episodes of depression at about the same age, and chronicity and recurrence are roughly equivalent for men and women. The gender difference first appears in adolescence, although rates are similar between girls and boys in childhood (Garrison, Addy, Jackson, McKeown, & Waller, 1992; Kandel & Davies, 1982; Lewinsohn, Hops, Roberts, Seeley, & Andrews, 1993), and in fact preadolescent boys are somewhat more prone to depression than preadolescent girls (Twenge & Nolen-Hoeksema, 2002).

Several interrelated hypotheses have been offered to account for gender differences. An early idea was that women and men actually experience depression at roughly equal rates, but that women are more likely to acknowledge and seek help for their depression, and in a related fashion, clinicians are more likely to overdiagnose depression in women than in men (Phillips & Segal, 1969). However, this artifact hypothesis has not received much empirical support. Another idea advanced to explain gender differences considers the role of precipitating events in onset of depression. Thus, women might be more likely to encounter traumatic events, childhood adversity, and interpersonal stressors. In general, data support each of these ideas (see Nolen-Hoeksema & Hilt, 2009), although the processes that create the transition between these problems and depression are not well understood.

Alternatively, biological hypotheses maintain that women are more vulnerable to depression because of endocrinological differences between men and women (Akiskal, 1987). A variety of specific ideas have been proposed that focus on changes associated with hormones, including the onset and timing of puberty (Angold & Costello, 1998), the menstrual cycle (Schmidt et al., 1991; Steiner, Dunn, & Born, 2003), menopause (Avis, 2003), and the postpartum period (Somerset et al., 2007). Evidence in each of these areas has been conflicting (Nolen-Hoeksema & Hilt, 2009), and thus despite a considerable amount of research, there is little uniform support for the view that hormones play a role in predisposing women to depression. Certainly it cannot be ruled out that hormonal differences may contribute to the higher incidence of depression in women, but how these processes contribute is far from clear. Likewise, genetic factors have been suggested to account for gender differences, but the evidence is far from clear as well (Lau & Eley, 2008).

Psychosocial factors have also been examined to account for gender differences in depression. Differences in interpersonal orientation represent one such idea, and suggest that women place greater value than men on friendships and relationships as sources of self-worth. However, relations can be fragile, and are dependent on others' behaviors, thus making women and their sense of self-worth susceptible to the uncontrollable vicissitudes of relationships. Certainly women and girls have been found to score higher than men and boys on measures of disproportionate concern with others (e.g., Nolen-Hoeksema & Jackson, 2001), and some evidence suggests that concerns about others' evaluations can mediate gender differences in depressive symptoms (e.g., Rudolph & Conley, 2005). There is thus promising evidence that differences in interpersonal orientation may play a role in gender differences.

Cognitive factors have been implicated in gender differences. For example, ruminative variables are suggested by cognitive models (e.g., those of Beck and Teasdale) to play an important role in depression, and some of the earliest work in the area found that women are more likely than men to ruminate (Nolen-Hoeksema, 1987) and focus their attention on themselves (Ingram, Cruet, Johnson, & Wisnicki, 1988). These types of cognitive processes have been linked to a variety of disordered states, including depression (Ingram, 1990). As Nolen-Hoeksema and Hilt (2009) note, "A greater tendency to ruminate may lead more women than men to cross the line from dysphoria to major depression, but once a woman (or man) has crossed that line, other processes may influence the duration of episodes" (p. 393). Such a process would explain the observation that women have more initial onsets of depression than men, but other variables (e.g., the length of depressive episodes) do not differ between the genders.

Although many of these ideas regarding gender differences in depression are plausible, and some combination of them are likely to account for these differences, none have yet to receive clear support (Nolen-Hoeksema & Hilt, 2009). Moreover, the study of gender differences has tended to ignore that fact that, while less commonly, men also get depressed. Hence models and data are needed to understand the processes that cause both men and women to become depressed, and of what accounts for these different rates.

Depression and Culture

We cannot do justice to the complexity of the all the issues involved in understanding depression across cultures. Indeed, despite more than 1,000 studies on culture over the last 15 years, Chentsova-Dutton and Tsai (2009) note that "it is sobering to realize how little we know about depression across cultures" (p. 378). *Culture* has many definitions, but can generally be thought of as a shared set of values, norms, and experiences that are tied to a particular nationality or ethnic group. Humans are arguably more alike than different, but these differences can play an important role in understanding depression. Culture can also be broken down within countries, so that in the United States, for example, Latino, African American, Asian American, Native American, and Caucasian groups share a national identity but also share within-group experiences. As we have noted, surveys of various groups tend to find few differences across the groups that are surveyed.

One issue that pervades considerations of depression and culture is the nature of the depression construct itself and how it might vary across cultures. In some cultures what might reflect depression is not expressed in ways that are in line with DSM-IV-TR definitions. In some non-Western cultures, there may be an absence of psychological components of depression and a dominance of somatic aspects (Marsella, Sartorius, Jablensky, & Fenton, 1985), which might not fit the definition of depression, despite the same underlying state. Responses to stress may also differ for different groups along both physiological and psychological lines. Rapidly changing political, social, and economic forces in some countries may also produce differences in depression, its associated features, or even what it looks like. Clearly, cultural variables are important in understanding depression, but the field appears to be far away from specifying these variables in their conceptual, empirical, and practical complexity.

Morbidity

Depression is associated with substantial impairment. Depressed individuals report substantially poorer intimate relationships and less satisfying social interactions than do members of the general population (Fredman, Weissman, Leaf, & Bruce, 1988). Depressed individuals also suffer severe health- and work-related disability. Wells et al. (1989) reported data suggesting that the impairment linked to depression is comparable to serious and chronic medical disorders. In another study, 23% of depressed individuals reported some days in which they were in bed all or most of the day in the previous 2 weeks, compared to only 5% of the general population (Wells, Golding, & Burnam, 1988). Likewise, 48% of depressed community respondents described their health as either poor or fair compared to 29% of those without depression (Well et al., 1989). Other research found that those with major depressive disorder reported 11 disability days per 90-day interval compared to 2.2 disability days for the general population (Broadhead et al., 1990). Given these data, it is not surprising that the amount of depression-related costs to the workplace is huge; Kessler et al. (2006) reported that the loss of productivity due to depression exceeds $36 billion annually when absenteeism and reduced job performance are factored in.

In addition to the cost to depressed people, depression can be costly to future generations as well. For example, the children of mothers with depression are at high risk for a range of problems, including psychopathology in general and depression in particular (Burbach & Borduin, 1986; Hammen, 2009). Studies have long suggested that children of depressed parents show deficits in academic performance, school behavior, and social competence (Rolf & Garmezy, 1974; Worland, Weeks, Janes, & Strock, 1984). Moreover, the children of depressed mothers do more poorly in social and academic spheres than do the children of psychiatrically normal women, or even of women with bipolar disorder or medically ill women (Anderson & Hammen, 1993).

Comorbidity

Depression is comorbid with a number of psychiatric and medical conditions. In the NCS-R findings, nearly 75% of those with lifetime depression also qualified for another psychiatric diagnosis (Kessler & Wang, 2009). Comorbidity is a significant problem, although it is also important to note that changes in the various editions of the DSM have contributed to multiple diagnoses. That is, beginning with DSM-III, many of the exclusionary criteria were dropped, making it possible for the individual who would have had one disorder according to earlier criteria to have more than one disorder with DSM-III or DSM-IV criteria. To provide a sense for the degree of comorbidity associated with depression according to DSM-IV-TR criteria, we briefly discuss some of the major issues of comorbidity and psychiatric disorders, medical disorders, and personality disorders.

Anxiety

Anxiety is one of the most common correlates of depression, although some of this co-occurrence may be accounted for by an overlap in diagnostic criteria; for example, difficulty concentrating, sleep disturbances, and fatigue appear in the diagnostic criteria for both major depressive disorder and generalized anxiety disorder. Even when diagnostic criteria overlap is taken into account, there is still substantial comorbidity between depressive and anxious states. In the NCS-R, 59% of people with a lifetime diagnosis of depression also met criteria for an anxiety disorder (Kessler et al., 2003). This finding is in line with a number of studies that have found either significant correlations between measures of depressive and anxious states, or the occurrence of a significant degree of anxiety in depressed individuals (and vice versa) (see Clark, 1989). Similarly, those with anxiety disorders frequently get depressed. Interestingly, it seems to be the case for many instances of comorbidity that the anxiety disorder preceded the depressive disorder.

Other Psychiatric Disorders

Schizophrenia is often associated with depression and, in fact, people diagnosed with schizophrenia have 28.5 times greater odds of being depressed than do nonschizophrenic individuals (Boyd et al., 1984). Similarly, many individuals with eating disorders also have symptoms of depression (Lewinsohn et al., 1993). Depression may be found in as many as 56% of individuals with anorexia (Hendren, 1983) and in approximately 24–33% of people with bulimia (Walsh, Roose, Glassman, Gladis, & Sadik, 1985). Although it is frequently unclear which disorder came first, there is no denying that significant psychopathology is often linked with depression.

Medical Disorders

In addition to psychiatric disorders, depression is also prevalent among patients with medical disorders. For instance, some research has found that approximately 4.8% to 9.2% of ambulatory medical patients have major depression (AHCPR Clinical Practice Guidelines, 1993). Depression also appears to be consistently linked to chronic medical conditions (Freedland & Carney, 2009). For example, data have shown a high degree of comorbidity between depression and both osteoarthritis and rheumatoid arthritis (Banks & Kerns, 1996; Romano & Turner, 1985; Smith, Wallston, & Dwyer, 1995).

The link between depression and medical illnesses can raise problems for both the clinical recognition of depression in medical patients, and for research seeking to examine depressive symptomatology in the context of medical illness. Like depression and anxiety, this problem pertains primarily to symptom overlap. For instance, if a cancer patient complains of loss of appetite, should this symptom be ascribed to the cancer or to depression, or to some combination of conditions? The depression symptoms that can frequently be correlates of medical illness include appetite/weight disturbance, psychomotor agitation/retardation, insomnia/hypersomnia, decreased libido, and fatigue. This is particularly true for chronic illness, and can substantially affect research results. For example, Peck, Smith, Ward, and Milano (1989) and Calfas, Ingram, and Kaplan (1997) found that the cognitive correlates of depression in chronic pain conditions are different when "depressive" symptoms are somatic in nature, and thus possibly the result of pain (e.g., difficulty sleeping, diminished enjoyment of activities), and are removed from diagnostic consideration. Thus, it may be that studies measuring only symptoms of depression and using cutoff scores established in healthy populations may overestimate psychiatric distress in medically ill patients.

Personality Disorders

Several important studies have examined the co-occurrence of personality disorders and depression. In the first, Shea, Glass, Pilkonis, Watkins, and Docherty (1987) found that, of a sample of 249 research participants, 75% persons with major depression had a definite or probably diagnosis of personality disorder. Likewise, Pilkonis and Frank (1988) found that 48% of a sample of patient with recurrent depression who had responded to treatment had concurrent probable or definite personality disorders. They found rates of co-occurrence were even higher for inpatients.

Comorbid personality disorder and depression has also been found to be related to decreased responsiveness to treatment of depression. That is, a number of studies have found that those depressed persons with personality disorders tend to do more poorly in both psychotherapy and pharmacotherapy interventions (e.g., Frank, Kupfer, Jacob, & Jarrett, 1987; Pilkonis & Frank, 1988). Clearly, the presence of a personality disorder, which is common, complicates depression.

Life Events

The impact of negative life events on depression has been well established (e.g., Monroe & Reid, 2009). Life stressors predict both the onset and maintenance of psychiatric distress, and events that involve significant loss, such as death of a spouse, are particularly likely to result in depression (Aneshensel, 1985; Billings, Cronkite, & Moos, 1983). Additionally, it has long been recognized that when negative life events occur, those that are uncontrollable are most strongly related to depression (McFarlane, Norman, Streiner, Roy, & Scott, 1980). Beyond acute stressors, chronic stressors including problems with finances, work, spouse, children, and physical health are also related to depression (Billings & Moos, 1982; Moos, Fenn, Billing, & Moos, 1989; Moos & Moos, 1992; Pearlin & Schooler, 1978; Revicki, Whitley, Gallery, & Allison, 1993).

It is easy to assume that the link between depression and stress moves in only one direction: stressors befall people, and that leads them to suffer depression. However, depressed individuals can also generate stress. Thus, for example, studies have found that chronically depressed people tend to experience more negative events as part of the social environment that they create and maintain (Hammen, 1991, 1992; Monroe, Kupfer, & Frank, 1992). More problematically, depression may generate stressful life events that in turn lead to continued depression (Coyne et al., 1987; Eberhart & Hammen, 2009).

SUMMARY

Much is known about the symptoms, characteristics, and features of depression as it is defined by DSM-IV-TR. Depending on different estimates, roughly 17% of the population has experienced a clinically severe episode of depression at some point in their lives, with women reporting approximately twice the rate as men. Depression in some form appears to exist in all cultures and subcultures, and is also comorbid with a number of other conditions. It is thus a pervasive disorder both in terms of its worldwide distribution and in terms of how it impairs functioning in a number of domains. However it is defined, what DSM refers to as depression represents a serious public health issue, which is evidenced by numerous theoretical, empirical, and clinical efforts to understand the disorder. We argue that a full understanding of depression must include the factors that place people at risk for depression. Such risk analyses are not only important for understanding the disorder, but can also inform efforts to treat and prevent depression. Before understanding vulnerability processes in depression, however, it is important to understand the assumptions that underlie vulnerability to depression. We turn to these assumptions and ideas next.

2

Why Vulnerability?

In this chapter we examine fundamental conceptual issues that apply to vulnerability. The focus of this chapter, however, is not on vulnerability to depression specifically, but instead provides an assessment of the construct as it pertains to psychopathology. We start by examining both the conceptual and the empirical origins of vulnerability. We next define vulnerability in reference to the idea that vulnerability is stable, endogenous, and latent. We also address the role of stress and the diathesis–stress link, and then conclude with an examination of several important issues in the study of vulnerability, such as the distinction between the ideas of risk and vulnerability.

ORIGINS OF THE VULNERABILITY APPROACH

To fully understand vulnerability it is helpful to understand the history and origins of the vulnerability concept. Thus, in the next two sections we address both the conceptual origins of the vulnerability construct (i.e., early theoretical approaches) and its empirical origins (i.e., early empirical findings).

Conceptual Origins: Schizophrenia

The origins of vulnerability applied to psychopathology are seen most clearly in the early work of schizophrenia theorists, most notably work by Meehl (1962) who was among the first to allude to a psychogenic vulnerability to the disorder. In his 1962 landmark paper, Meehl proposed that the onset of a schizophrenic episode is dependent on neural deficits, labeled "schizotaxia," as well as on the individual's particular learning history, a combination that he referred to as "schizotypia." Schizotypia in and of itself, however, was not considered to be sufficient to precipitate a schizophrenic episode. Meehl suggested that only some schizotypic individuals would eventually decompensate into clinical schizophrenia, a subset determined by the presence of a schizophrenogenic mother who exposed the child to a developmental climate of unpredictable, ambivalent, and aversive mother–child interactions: "It seems likely that the most important causal influence pushing the schizotype toward schizophrenic decompensation is the schizophrenogenic mother" (p. 830). Meehl therefore suggested that the onset of clinical schizophrenia was a function of vulnerability factors that were both genetic and psychogenic. It is also worth noting that by describing the importance of the unpredictable and aversive mother–child interactions Meehl brought together the idea of vulnerability and stress interaction.

Since the publication of Meehl's seminal paper, several investigators have alluded to various schizophrenia vulnerability possibilities (e.g., Gottesman & Shields, 1972; Millon, 1969). Among the first to explicitly discuss vulnerability were Zubin and Spring (1977), who argued that research progress on the causes of schizophrenia was at best equivocal and that investigators were generally dissatisfied with the adequacy of the major conceptual approaches to the etiology of the disorder (e.g., environmental, genetic, developmental, neurophysiological). To resolve this problem, they suggested that vulnerability could be viewed as a common denominator underlying all of the conceptual approaches to schizophrenia. Thus, although the major etiological models emphasized different approaches, all share the possibility that some vulnerability factor might predispose the person to the development of a schizophrenic episode.

Considering the various etiological perspectives on schizophrenia as well as the suggestions of other researchers who had anticipated the vulnerability idea (e.g., Gottsman & Shields, 1972; Meehl, 1962; Millon, 1969; Rosenthal, 1970), Zubin and Spring (1977) proposed that vulnerability consisted of both acquired and genetic factors that they phrased as "acquired and inborn":

> Inborn vulnerability [is] that which is laid down in the genes and reflected in the internal environment and neurophysiology of the organism. The acquired component of vulnerability is due to the influence of traumas, specific diseases, perinatal complications, family

experiences, adolescent peer interactions, and other life events that either enhance or inhibit the development of subsequent disorder. (p. 109)

Zubin and Spring (1977) also hypothesized that people's coping efforts (e.g., "the energy exerted in situations") and competence (e.g., "the skills and abilities needed to achieve success") are involved in the initiation of a schizophrenic episode. Competence and coping efforts together comprise a person's coping *ability*, "the initiative and skill that an organism brings to bear in formulating strategies to master life situations" (p. 123). Zubin and Spring, however, argued that although coping ability is important, it operates independently of vulnerability factors. Specifically, they suggested that even though some data show that competence is low during a schizophrenic episode, research is unclear as to whether competence deficiencies are due to premorbid competence deficits or are instead a function of life stress and disorder-induced strains that decrease the competence level. Although coping ability and vulnerability were seen as distinct, Zubin and Spring noted the possibility of an indirect link; they suggested that people whose coping has been compromised were more likely to experience exacerbated stress and therefore heightened risk for disorder.

Conceptual Origins: The Diathesis–Stress Perspective

Aside from a focus on schizophrenia, what Meehl (1962) and Zubin and Spring (1977) also share is a focus on a diathesis–stress perspective in understanding the onset of psychopathology. *Diathesis* is traditionally defined as a predisposition to a disorder, and depending on the particular model, can encompass genetic, biological, social, behavioral, and psychological factors. Irrespective of the particular level of analysis, the onset of psychopathology, in this case schizophrenia, is viewed as a function of the interactive effect of the diatheses together with events perceived as stressful. As we will see, diathesis–stress approaches also play a vital role in understanding depression.

Conceptual Origins: Beyond Schizophrenia

Schizophrenia investigators were the first, but not the only, investigators who recognized the potential usefulness of the vulnerability construct. Developmental psychopathologists, for instance, have focused considerable attention on factors that may either predispose or insulate children from psychological problems. The list includes psychological disorders, behavioral difficulties, academic performance deficits, and interpersonal problems (e.g., Rutter, 1988). Likewise, alcoholism (Pollock et al., 1988), bipolar disorder (Depue et al., 1981), and psychopathy (Kandel et al., 1988; Widom, 1977) all represent psychopathological states that have been the focus of vulnerability analyses, and in many cases also incorporate diathesis–stress frameworks.

Empirical Origins of the Vulnerability Construct

A number of relatively early empirical studies relied on vulnerability perspectives, but did so without a clearly articulated vulnerability perspective; that is, researchers recognized vulnerability when they saw it, even if the concept had not yet been fully defined for a particular disorder. Examining this research can help pinpoint some of the origins of this perspective. A number of approaches for empirically identifying and studying vulnerable individuals have been employed, all of which will be discussed more in depth later in this book, and so here we provide a brief overview of some strategies focused on identifying vulnerable individuals.

A common strategy for identifying potentially vulnerable individuals is to assess the offspring of parents with a psychological disorder, a strategy that is frequently referred to as the *high-risk paradigm*. The assumption guiding many investigators using this strategy is that, presumably through either genetic or environmental influences, offspring are at risk for developing disorders similar to their parents' disorders. This is again illustrated in efforts to understand schizophrenia. For example, studies reported by Mednick and Schulsinger (1968), Kety, Rosenthal, Wender, and Schulsinger (1968), and Rosenthal et al. (1968) assessed a number of variables in the offspring of a parent (or parents) with a diagnosis of schizophrenia. Using extensive registers in Denmark known as the National Psychiatric Register and the Folkeregister, these investigators were able to locate a large number of offspring of Danish schizophrenic mothers. The Folkeregister is an up-to-date register of the addresses of virtually every resident of Denmark, and the National Psychiatric Register maintains a record of all psychiatric hospitalizations in Denmark. Mednick and Schulsinger (1968) used these databases to locate a sample of 207 children of schizophrenic mothers and a control group of 104 healthy children. Data were collected on a number of variables and the sample was followed over a period of time. Few investigators, however, have the luxury of access to such comprehensive databases.

Beyond schizophrenia, this strategy is nicely illustrated by Klein, Depue, and Krauss's (1986) assessment of social adjustment as a possible risk variable in the children of parents with bipolar disorder, and Walker and Hoppes's (1984) review of the impact of parental schizophrenia on offspring. In regard to depression, Hammen's (2009) and Goodman's (e.g., Goodman, 2007; Goodman & Tully, 2008) work examining a number of factors in the children of depressed mothers is a comprehensive illustration of the high-risk strategy, and has provided comprehensive review of research employing the strategy of assessing the effects of maternal depression on offspring.

Some researchers have sought other ways to identify and investigate individuals vulnerable to psychopathology. For instance, another strategy is to identify high-risk individuals on the basis of some theoretical or empirical criterion. Using such a strategy, Depue, Krauss, Spoont, and Arbisi (1989), for example, identified individuals vulnerable to clinical bipolar disorder based on their responses on self-report questionnaires designed to assess factors hypothesized to reflect risk for the disorder. Investigators, once they have identified individuals in this fashion, investigators can attempt to elicit evidence for the existence of increased risk for psychopathology.

DEFINING VULNERABILITY

As we noted, clinicians and researchers know vulnerability when they see it, but few have proposed precise definitions of the construct. This is not a problem to the public in general in that the concept of vulnerability is easily defined; people are vulnerable to the extent that they are susceptible to, or more likely than others to, being hurt or wounded. Extension of this definition to psychological domains implies an increased susceptibility to emotional pain and to the occurrence of psychopathology of some type. Yet, as intuitively appealing as this concept is, more precise definitions of vulnerability are needed if clinicians and researchers are to make progress in comprehensively understanding psychopathology in general and depression in particular. We argue that the best way of defining vulnerability is by noting the core features of the concept.

Core Features of Vulnerability

As is evident from the preceding discussion, the vulnerability approach to psychopathology is at least several decades old. Yet, as we have noted, as widespread as this approach is there are few precise definitions of vulnerability in the literature. Despite this fact, it is possible to garner from previous theory and research the core characteristics of the construct. Such characteristics generally constitute the common themes that emerge in discussions of vulnerability and can thus help establish a consensus for what vulnerability is, and what it is not.

Vulnerability Is Stable

Most discussions of vulnerability regard it as a trait. Zubin and Spring (1977) may have articulated this idea the best: "We regard [vulnerability] as a relatively permanent, enduring trait" (p. 109); "The one feature that all schizophrenics have ... is the everpresence of their vulnerability" (p. 122). Although other investigators may not have been quite as specific, the enduring trait nature of vulnerability is implicit in their discussions of vulnerability, and are undoubtedly rooted in the genetic level of analysis employed by the researchers who pioneered this concept. Indeed, many schizophrenia researchers point to the genetic characteristics of individuals who are at risk for this disorder. For example, Meehl's (1962) concept of schizotaxia reflects an inherited neural deficit, whereas other researchers are explicit in claiming that genetic endowment plays an important role in creating vulnerability (at least to schizophrenia) (e.g., Nicholson & Neufeld, 1992; Zubin & Spring, 1972). Significant change is not theoretically possible; genetic endowment, and hence vulnerability, is seen as permanent.

Although these conceptualizations posit that no decrease in absolute vulnerability levels is possible, *functional* vulnerability levels may be affected by several factors, such as those that affect neurochemistry. By presumably controlling the neurochemistry of the underlying vulnerability, this may very well be the case for pharmacological interventions. However, although functional vulnerability may be altered and the individual is less likely to develop the disorder, the vulnerability persists; in the case of lithium for bipolar disorder, for example, a high probability of developing an episode occurs when medication is discontinued. Therefore, even though the risk may be controlled, the underlying vulnerability itself remains.

The enduring nature of vulnerability can clearly be seen in contrast to the state or episodic nature of psychological disorders. For instance, Zubin and Spring (1977) draw a clear distinction between enduring vulnerability and episodes of schizophrenia which "are waxing and waning states" (p. 109). Likewise, Hollon, Evans, and DeRubeis (1990) and Hollon and Cobb (1993) distinguish between (1) stable vulnerability characteristics that predispose individuals to the disorder but do not initiate the disorder, and (2) state variables representing symptoms that reflect the onset of the disorder. Hence, investigators characterize the disorder as a state and see predisposing factors as traits. Disordered states therefore emerge and fade as episodes cycle between occurrence and remission, but the vulnerability traits that give rise to the disordered state are typically thought to be unchanging.

Even though vulnerability is assumed by many theorists to be permanent and unchanging, this need not always be the case. As we have noted, assumptions of genetic risk suggest little possibility for modification of vulnerability. Most psychological approaches to risk, however, rely on assumptions of dysfunctional learning as the genesis of vulnerability. Given such assumptions, not only functional but actual vulnerability levels may change as a function of new learning experiences. For instance, Hollon et al. (2006) review data suggesting that depressed patients treated with cognitive therapy, or combined cognitive therapy and pharmacotherapy, are less likely than patients treated with pharmacotherapy alone to experience recurrence of the disorder over a 2-year period. Hollon et al. (1990) and Hollon and Cobb (1993) argue that the effects of pharmacological treatments may "simply" suppress symptoms, whereas psychological interventions like cognitive therapy appear to alter depressive cognitive structures (Garratt, Ingram, Rand, & Sawalani, 2007). To the extent that vulnerability is rooted in such structures, vulnerability to future depression is decreased or in some cases eliminated.

Of course, from the viewpoint of psychological analyses, vulnerability may *decrease* with certain corrective experiences, but it may also *increase* over time; we elaborate in more detail on this possibility in the discussion of diathesis–stress models. For now we note that it could be the case that continued exposure to aversive experiences and stressful life events serve to exacerbate the factors that contribute to vulnerability. From a cognitive viewpoint this would be seen in experiences that increased the complexity and accessibility of dysfunctional cognitive self-structures.

Permanence versus Stability

The possibility that psychological vulnerability levels can be altered suggests a subtle but potentially important distinction between stability and permanence. Although stability and permanence are likely to be viewed as synonymous with one another, the concept of stability in fact suggests a resistance to change—it does not presume that change is never possible. Under the optimal circumstances, changes in an otherwise stable variable may very well occur, and, indeed, the notion of psychotherapy is based on just this premise. Without significant life experiences, or psychotherapy, however, little change in stable variables should be seen. Variables that are considered to be enduring (e.g., particularly as viewed within a genetic context) suggest a permanence or immutability that is not only resistant to change under ordinary circumstances, but is in fact assumed to offer virtually no possibility of change. At the psychological level of analysis, then, it seems reasonable to conceptualize vulnerability as stable, and possibly resistant to change but not absolutely immutable.

Vulnerability Is Endogenous

Another idea that is possible to glean from extant vulnerability work is that vulnerability represents an endogenous process. This is clearly seen in genetic conceptualizations of vulnerability, but is equally relevant for psychological conceptualizations. That is, whether stemming from biological processes, inborn characteristics, or acquired-through-learning processes, the vulnerability process resides within the person. This can be contrasted to other viewpoints that might focus on environmental or external sources that initiate a disorder, or perhaps that focus on certain interactional styles and dynamics (e.g., Coyne, 1976; Joiner & Coyne, 1999). Clearly, such variables are important, but vulnerability itself is seen as emanating from within the person.

Vulnerability Is Latent

Vulnerability researchers frequently categorize vulnerability as a latent process that is not easily observable. This can perhaps be seen most clearly in the empirical search for observable markers of vulnerability; numerous investigators have sought to find reliable indicators of the presence of theorized risk mechanisms. A variety of research strategies for identifying such processes have been used, which tend to operate under the assumptions that (1) vulnerability processes are present in individuals who have few or no outward signs of the disorder, (2) they are causally linked to the appearance of symptoms, and (3) they are not easily observable. This is particularly true for investigations that rely on some kind of stressful or challenging event that makes detection of the vulnerability factor possible (see Shelton, Hollon, Purdon, & Loosen, 1991, for a discussion of such challenge paradigms as they pertain to the conceptualization of vulnerability and dysregulation). The search for vulnerability variables is thus the search for predictors of the disorder in the absence of symptoms of the disorder, an empirical strategy reflecting a conceptual judgment that vulnerability is present and stable, but latent.

The Role of Stress

Owing to our assumption that vulnerability is endogenous, stress cannot be considered to be part of vulnerability. While technically true, however, to fully understand the nature of vulnerability, we must also understand the role of stress. We therefore consider stress as a necessary factor in any definition of vulnerability.

Stress has been defined in such a diversity of ways that to comprehensively examine these definitions would necessitate an entire book. And indeed entire books have been devoted to this topic, from classic work (e.g., Brown & Harris, 1989; Cohen, 1988; Lazarus & Folkman, 1984) to more recent work (Kalueff & La Porte, 2008). For our purposes, we can think of stress as falling into two broad categories. The first major category of stress refers to the occurrence of significant life events that are interpreted as undesirable and the second is seen as the accumulation of minor events or hassles (e.g., Dohrenwend & Shrout, 1985; Lazarus, 1990). Alternatively, a number of investigators (e.g., Luthar & Zigler, 1991; Monroe, 2008; Monroe & Simons, 1991) focus more on the occurrence of significant life events. We can therefore view stress as the life events (major or minor) that disrupt the stability of physiology, emotion, and cognition. In the classic and still relevant description of stress, Selye (1936) argues that such events represent a strain on adaptive capacity that causes interruptions of the person's routine or habitual functioning. In this view, stress disrupts the system's psychological and physiological homeostasis and, as such, has been incorporated as a critical variable in numerous models of psychopathology (Monroe & Reid,

2009; Monroe & Simons, 1991), regardless of whether or not these models focus explicitly on vulnerability factors.

As we have alluded to, stress is typically seen as reflecting factors operating outside of, or externally to, the individual; they are the life events that challenge the person's coping resources. An external orientation does not mean, however, that individuals play no role in creating stress. That is, although there are events that befall people (independent events), several researchers have persuasively argued that some stressful events are the result of a person's own actions (dependent events) (Depue & Monroe, 1986; Hammen, 1991; Monroe & Reid, 2009; Monroe & Simons, 1991). For example, the person with social skills deficits (e.g., someone who is inappropriately critical of others) may engender tumultuous relationships with acquaintances, coworkers, and romantic partners that result in the generation of stress. It thus is possible that vulnerable individuals may play a role in creating their own stresses that may then precipitate psychological disorder.

In addition to the complexities ensuing from the recognition that stress can be generated by individuals, investigators have pointed out that it is notoriously difficult to disentangle external stress from cognitive appraisal processes. This is particularly the case for individuals who are thought to be vulnerable to or are in a psychologically disordered state (Lazarus & Folkman, 1984; Monroe & Simons, 1991). For example, the person experiencing significant anxiety may perceive relatively safe events as posing considerable physical or psychological danger, thus evaluating events as stressful. Along these lines, Nicholson and Neufeld (1992) have argued that vulnerability affects the perceptions of stress, even genetically based vulnerability; they note that "genetic makeup affects cognitive appraisal mechanisms, partly determining how accurately the individual is able to assess a [stressful] situation" (p. 122).

The influence of appraisal processes on the perception of stress has created significant methodological difficulties for the objective measurement of stress (Monroe, 1989; Monroe & Simons, 1991). Other problems also exist, such as distinguishing between stressful events that precede and are perhaps linked to the onset of symptomatology, from those that follow and are the result of a disorder. That is, rather than stress precipitating the disorder, it may be that the disorder precipitates the experience of negative life events. Distinguishing which came first is a methodological challenge.

Some investigators have argued that to even attempt to separate stress from a person's life at all is artificial; life events and lifestyle are intrinsically related (Kasl, 1983). Moreover, assessing the timing of stressful events as they relate to disorder can also be problematic. What is the "correct" time frame by which investigators can link stress and psychopathology? Are, for example, stressful life events that precede a disorder by 2 years (1 month, 12 months, 5 years?) related to the onset of the disorder, and how can this causal connection be empirically confirmed?

Clearly, the problems with the conceptualization and measurement of stressful events are extensive. Stress and disorder can be so closely interwoven that it makes little sense to try to separate them. Nevertheless, we argue that at a conceptual level it does make sense to separate stress from vulnerability and from psychological disorder. Such a conceptual separation recognizes the possibility that stress can exist independently of psychopathology and appraisal processes, and can be consensually defined and objectively measured. Everyone would agree, for example, that a car accident resulting in permanent confinement to a wheel chair will be stressful for everyone regardless of appraisal processes. Moreover, separating the stress and vulnerability constructs facilitates communication; that is, it is possible to talk about stress without frequent qualifications due to appraisal processes. Perhaps the most important reason for separating these variables is that it allows us to conceptually talk about how they are connected in bringing about the onset of psychopathology, specifically, to talk about the diathesis–stress idea.

The Diathesis–Stress Association

The idea of a diathesis has a long history in medical terminology. In tracing this history, for example, Monroe and Simons (1991) note that the concept dates back to the ancient Greeks, and that as early as the late 1800s the term was already established in psychiatry. *Diathesis* refers to a risk or a predisposition to illness, and has evolved from its original focus on constitutional and biological factors to currently also encompass psychological variables. In line with this idea, many, if not most, psychological models of depression and vulnerability are explicitly diathesis–stress models. Specifically, while there is general agreement in the field that vulnerability constitutes an endogenous process, it is also recognized that stressful events act to trigger vulnerability processes that are linked to the onset of depression.

Given the importance of the diathesis–stress relationship in psycho-pathology in general and depression in particular, it is worth exploring some of the attributes of this relationship, and the different forms that the relationship can take. That is, a variety of diathesis–stress models have been proposed for various types of psychopathology (see Ingram & Price, 2010), yet there are differences in the structures of diathesis–stress conceptualizations. Once such structure emphasizes that additive nature of diathesis and stress processes in the production of produce psychopathology.

ADDITIVITY MODELS

On the surface, diathesis–stress models represent a linear dose–response relationship. At the most basic level, this idea suggests that the development of a disorder depends on the combined effects of stress and the loading of the diathesis. A model may suggest, for example, that even very minor stressors will precipitate the onset of the disorder for a person who is highly vulnerable, and would correspondingly suggest that a major stressful event might cause a similar reaction in a person low in vulnerability. Alternatively, a model might suggest that both a significant degree of vulnerability and a significant amount of stress are needed to trigger a disorder. For the sake of simplicity, Ingram and Luxton (2005) termed this a *mega* diathesis–stress model to denote that both the diathesis and the stress must be considerable before a disorder occurs. Although different models may accord a stronger role for one component or the other, this idea suggests additivity, that diatheses and stress add together in some way to produce the disorder.

IPSATIVE MODELS

Ipsative models are not necessarily distinct from additive approaches, but offer somewhat greater specificity in describing the diathesis–stress relationship. In particular, ipsative models specify an inverse relationship between factors: the greater the presence of one factor, the less of the other factor is needed to bring about the disorder (Monroe & Hadjiyannakis, 2002). Thus, the degree of effect of diathesis or stress can be offset or compensated by the other in the summation that is needed for psychopathology. Like additivity models, however, these models suggest that the diathesis and the stress sum together to cause psychopathology.

DYNAMIC AND STATIC DIATHESIS–STRESS RELATIONSHIPS

Examination of these models reveals a neglected aspect of many diathesis–stress models of psychopathology, specifically the distinction between the idea that the nature of the diathesis–stress relationship does not change, or changes little, versus the idea that the relationship between the diathesis and the stress can change over time (Monroe & Harkness, 2005). As Monroe and Harkness (2005) note, this changing interaction can be illustrated by reference to the idea of kindling (see Post, 1992, 2007). *Kindling* suggests that repeated instances of disorder cause neuronal changes that result in more sensitivity to stress. Kindling accounts for the fact that first episodes of depression are more strongly interlinked to the experience of stress than are subsequent episodes (Post, 2009). Although some have suggested that over time these processes become delinked completely, and that episodes of depression than occur "autonomously," a viable alternative to this idea is that with heightened vulnerability, less stress becomes necessary to activate depression (Monroe & Harkness, 2005). Thus while stress may become more difficult to detect, it is still present and serves to elicit an episode, such as the case of the women whose depression is triggered by her favorite TV show being cancelled. This idea suggests that the association between diatheses and stress is not necessarily static, and more specifically, that processes involved may become more ipsative. That is, while a mega model suggests that high levels of both stress and diatheses are needed, a heightened sensitivity leads to an inverted link wherein diatheses are strengthened so that less stress becomes necessary to activate depression.

Summary of Core Features of Vulnerability

In sum, several essential features characterize the construct of vulnerability. Perhaps the most fundamental feature of vulnerability is that it is considered a trait as opposed to the kind of a state that more accurately characterizes a psychopathological episode. However, even though vulnerability is conceptualized as a stable characteristic, psychologically construed vulnerability may be stable and relatively resistant to change, but it is not necessarily permanent. Continued exposure to aversive experiences may increase vulnerability factors, or alternatively, corrective experiences can occur that attenuate the vulnerability. Additionally, vulnerability is seen as a latent and endogenous process, and although stress is conceptually distinct from vulnerability, it is nevertheless a critical "feature" of vulnerability in that vulnerability cannot be realized without stress.

IMPORTANT ISSUES IN THE STUDY OF VULNERABILITY

Having examined some of the core features that comprise a definition of vulnerability, we now turn to a general discussion of several conceptual issues that are important to consider in the study of this idea as applied to depression. In particular, we address psychological conceptualizations of vulnerability analyses, the relationship between risk and vulnerability, and the relationship between vulnerability and resilience.

The Analysis of Vulnerability from a Psychological Perspective

Much of the original work we have reviewed to provide a foundation for the vulnerability perspective has focused on vulnerability at the genetic level (e.g., schizotypia). "Acquired" factors have tended to be secondary in these models, but even these factors are apt to be viewed from a biological viewpoint. Zubin and Spring (1977), for instance, describe some of these acquired factors as "the influence of traumas, specific diseases, [and] perinatal complications" (p. 109) that presumably affect the biochemistry of those who thus become vulnerable to schizophrenia. Acquired factors, however, need not be limited to biochemical levels of analysis; they can also refer to learned processes (e.g., a learning climate of ambivalence brought about by a schizophrenogenic mother) that are acknowledged even in some predominantly genetic models to play an important, albeit secondary, contributory role in vulnerability.

Accounts of vulnerability that are primarily psychological are, of course, bound by biology, but emphasize that acquired variables are, in the broadest sense of the term, learned. Such variables are quite diverse, ranging from a focus on the person's competence and coping in difficult circumstances to variables such as maternal ambivalence and disrupted early interpersonal relationships. In the former case, for example, vulnerability may in fact be a direct function of coping processes; those who experience stressful life events but who cannot effectively manage them may in fact be vulnerable because of (presumably learned) coping deficits.

All of these types of processes (e.g., coping deficits, maternal ambivalence, interpersonal disruptions) are thought to either affect how and what people learn, or are considered to be the result of some learning process. These types of factors reflect fundamental variables in many psychological analyses of mental disorders. We note the relevance of these variables to contrast them from models that specifically rule out psychological factors as meaningful vulnerability variables.

The Relationship between Risk and Vulnerability

To the extent that any variable can be shown to be related to an increased probability of disorder onset, the variable can be considered to be a risk factor. Any number of variables can describe people as being "at risk" for a psychopathological state such as depression. To illustrate this point, Kaelber, Moul, and Farmer (1995) summarized a multitude of potential risk factors for the occurrence of depression and distinguished between risk indicators that are (1) highly plausible, (2) plausible, and (3) possible. Factors such as being female, experiencing depression in the past, being divorced or separated, living in low socioeconomic circumstances, and having smoked are listed in the highly plausible category, while in the plausible category factors include losing a mother before age 11, being never married, having a family history of depression, and having small children at home. Among others in the possible category are living in a city, chronically doing housework, being infertile, or being a Protestant. Indeed, the sheer number and breath of demonstrated risk factors is quite impressive.

Even though possessing a risk factors suggest an enhanced probability of disorder, and it is therefore important to examine these factors, risk factors in and of themselves are relatively uninformative about an individual's vulnerability—that is, they do not tell us about the actual *mechanisms* that bring about a state of psychopathology. While being a city-living, divorced, Protestant who smokes while doing housework might suggest ideas about the onset of depression, there is nothing inherent in these risk characteristics that causes depression. Likewise, knowledge of such risk indicators is generally unhelpful with regard to specific intervention strategies. Changing religions (and even gender) is possible, as is refraining from housework and quitting smoking, but these changes do not directly influence vulnerability to depression.

We note these issues about the idea of risk because the terms "risk" and "vulnerability" are often used interchangeably. Certainly these ideas share substantial conceptual variance, but risk and vulnerability are dif-

ferent constructs. While risk describes factors that are statistically associated with an increased likelihood of experiencing a disorder, vulnerability refers to the mechanisms that bring about a disorder. Hence, if
depression is rooted in the dysregulation of a certain neurotransmitter,
then this variable constitutes a vulnerability factor. Or, if depression is
precipitated by the activation of schemas that influence how information
is processed, these schemas and their activation constitute vulnerability
factors. Vulnerability factors are thus presumed to be causal factors. Of
course, given the definition of risk, vulnerability factors must also constitute risk factors—that is, possessing vulnerability also places one at
risk. Vulnerability is therefore most properly seen as a subset of risk, and
as such, risk conceptually comprises a much broader network of factors
than does vulnerability.

In noting a similar separation between risk and vulnerability Rutter
(1987) and Luthar and Zigler (1991) also discuss how risk variables can
predict the onset of psychopathology, and how they tend to be correlated with vulnerability. Although these associations may make it tempt-
ing to suggest that risk has causal significance, Rutter (1988) specifically
cautions against drawing casual inferences solely from risk variables
that appear linked to a disorder. In particular, he notes that risk and
vulnerability are correlated by virtue of their interaction in the onset of
psychopathology. To illustrate, Rutter (1988) notes findings from his
research showing that test results on a national examination were superior for schools where the children's work was displayed on the school
walls (i.e., Rutter, Maughan, Mortimore, & Ouston, 1979). This variable, exhibiting artworks, empirically constitutes a predictor of better
test performance, but no one would argue that putting children's work
on a wall helped their test grades, that it was the casual factor in getting
better grades. Rather, displaying artwork was more likely to be predictive of an enhanced school atmosphere that was the causal link to better
performance. Likewise, the fact that being unmarried predicts psychopathology does not suggest that it causes psychopathology; it may be
predicative for a number of reasons. For instance, the unmarried man's
self-esteem may be so deficient that he is unable to initiate or maintain
romantic relationships that would eventuate in marriage. If this deficient
self-esteem is the causal (i.e., vulnerability) factor, then being unmarried
may predict psychopathology, but is a correlate rather than a cause. In
sum, then, risk can be an important predictive variable that can act in
concert with vulnerability, but clearly vulnerability and risk are not the
same.

The Relationship between Resilience and Vulnerability

A number of terms have been used by various investigators to label the flip side of vulnerability: "invulnerability," "competence," "protective factors," "resilience." Each of these terms suggests a resistance to psychopathology in the face of stress. Although in some cases these terms may reasonably be used interchangeably, subtle differences in their meaning also suggest distinctions between terms. For instance, "invulnerability" suggests people are either vulnerable or they are invulnerable, with little possibility of a state in between; that is, to the extent that individuals are invulnerable, this implies that they will never experience a disorder. Additionally, we believe that competence is too broad a term to describe the opposite of vulnerability (e.g., it can be used to refer to behavioral competence, such as one's ability to successfully complete a task).

Referring to the opposite of vulnerability in terms of protective factors raises important empirical issues that have not yet been resolved. Specifically, protective factors imply the presence of processes that actively protect against disorder. This idea, however, can be contrasted with the possibility that resistance to a disorder consists of the absence of vulnerability factors rather than to the presence of protective factors. Of course, some combination is also possible: the absence of some vulnerability processes along with the presence of some protective factors. For all of these reasons, we prefer the term "resilience" over others because it implies a diminished, but not zero, possibility of psychopathology, and does not assume the presence of as yet unknown variables.

Few empirical data have been reported that explore the relationship between vulnerability and resilience. Our working assumption, however, is that resilience and vulnerability represent different ends of a continuum. The variables on this continuum are seen as interacting with stress to produce the possibility that a disordered state will occur. Thus, at the vulnerability end of the range, relatively little life stress is necessary to produce a disorder, whereas at the resilient end of the range a great deal of stress is needed before psychopathology develops.

The vulnerability–resilience relationship is depicted in Figure 2.1. As this figure shows, as resilience decreases the probability that stress will result in a disorder increases. At the other end, as resilience increases, the risk for disorder goes down, but does not disappear entirely. Thus, with sufficient stress, even the most resilient of people will be at risk for the development of symptoms that would permit a diagnosis, although these symptoms and the diagnosis they represent will probably be milder

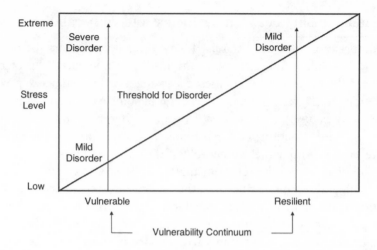

FIGURE 2.1. Relationship between vulnerability, resilience, stress, and disorder.

than that of the vulnerable person who experiences low to moderate stress, and almost certainly milder than the vulnerable person under significant stress. While intended to apply to depression, this framework may reflect other instances of psychopathology. For instance, Zubin and Spring (1977) suggest that under significant stress even resilient individuals may experience "mini-episodes" of psychosis, albeit briefer and less intense than those experienced by vulnerable persons. Moreover, official classification systems also recognize that otherwise resilient people can experience symptomatology with enough stress. Resilience therefore suggests the converse of vulnerability and implies a resistance to disorder, but not a complete immunity to disorder.

Conceptions of Causality

Although the ideas of onset and maintenance are fundamental to any understanding of depression, some researchers tacitly identify the onset or appearance of depressive symptomatology as synonymous with the factors that cause depression. And, because they are not viewed as causal, relatively little importance is given to the factors that help maintain the state. Causality, however, is not synonymous with onset and we thus believe this to be too narrow a conception of the construct of causality. By virtually all estimates, depression is a persistent disorder with symptoms lasting months (sometimes even with effective treatment), and in some cases years. Indeed, the symptoms that endure over a long period of time are most likely linked to the disruption and personal turmoil that accompany depression. Thus, the factors involved in the perpetuation of depression can be considered to have very real casual significance. We can thus ask whether the maintenance aspect of causality is any less important than causality viewed in terms of onset perspectives. From the standpoint of understanding the causes of depression, the distinction between onset and maintenance may be more artificial than it is genuinely helpful.

A related issue to understanding causality is the ability of research designs to demonstrate causation, whether from an onset or a maintenance prospective. Causality is notoriously difficult to demonstrate, even if a variable is shown to predict the occurrence, or perpetuation, of depression. It may be, for example, that correlated with studied variables are other variables that in reality serve as the causative factors for depression. Thus, even though demonstrating that some variables predict depression is an important step, issues of third variable causality cannot be ruled out.

SUMMARY: TOWARD A GENERAL CONCEPTUALIZATION OF VULNERABILITY

In this chapter we noted that the idea of vulnerability is relatively recent in the psychological literature, and originated first with Meehl's (1962) discussion of the role that both biological and psychological factors play in schizophrenia. Like the conceptual origins of vulnerability, its empirical origins can also be traced to studies of individuals at risk for schizophrenia, which subsequently paved the way for the empirical examination of vulnerability to a variety of disorders.

We also examined the core features that characterize many of the assumptions about the nature of vulnerability. Given these features, what can we regard as a reasonable definition of vulnerability? For one, vulnerability is seen as a stable characteristic, but we also noted that stability does not imply permanence. That is, at least, under some circumstances, vulnerability levels may be altered in either positive or negative ways. Second, the stable nature of this construct suggests that vulnerability be viewed as residing internally. Vulnerability is different than risk, and risk can include external factors. Vulnerability, however, is also a risk factor, suggesting that it is a subcategory of the broader idea of risk.

Third, vulnerability is distinct from the symptoms of the disorder; in most psychological models of disorder, symptoms are brought about by the interaction between stressful events and the presence of a vulnerability factor. In this sense, vulnerability serves as the final common pathway by which a broad array of risk factors (e.g., stress) lead to a disorder, and thus does so in the context of a diathesis–stress model. Moreover, the diathesis–stress idea illustrates that vulnerability is latent, suggesting that evidence of vulnerability can be difficult to detect without eliciting conditions. This idea thus requires investigators to specify the conditions under which vulnerability can be detected (Hollon, 1992; Segal & Ingram, 1994), an idea that we address later in this book.

In sum, then, vulnerability can be defined as a stable and internal feature of the person that predisposes him or her to the development of psychopathology when stressful life events occur. There are, of course, individuals who are resistant to the deleterious effects of such events, which we view as resilience, although resilience does not imply immunity. Having proposed a broad definition of vulnerability, we now turn to an examination of methodological issues and strategies in the study of vulnerability.

3

Cognitive–Clinical Science and Cognitive Neuroscience Approaches to Understanding Behavior

Our focus in this volume is to examine risk from the complementary approaches offered by cognitively oriented clinical psychology and by cognitive neuroscience. Prior to doing so, we discuss a number of elements concerning these approaches. We start with an examination of the guiding assumptions of cognitive–clinical science and then discuss the recent historical background of this approach. We note also the evolution from information-processing ideas to ideas informed by cognitive neuroscience and then examine some of the basic ideas in neuroscience, concluding with a discussion of neuroscience models of emotion.

Before we examine these conceptual approaches and their origins, it is important to consider how cognitive neuroscience and cognitive–clinical science are, and are not, related. We discuss the areas of divergence and convergence in more detail in Chapter 7, but note here that these approaches, despite their differences, are well matched with one another. That is, they focus on similar phenomena and have similar goals, with cognitive neuroscience tackling the "brain part" of the puzzle and cognitive–clinical science taking the "mind part." Hence, there are crucial compatibilities between these perspectives, and current knowledge garnered from both of these areas has brought about a better understanding of depression and depression vulnerability, and, as we will see, of the treatment of these problems. Hopefully these different viewpoints will eventually lead to a more complete integration of theoretical ideas about risk for depression.

Even though cognitive–clinical science and cognitive neuroscience are complementary, it is important to recognize their differences and the limitations of each. For instance, while the phenomena they investigate are similar, the methods they use, and what is possible to learn from these methods, tends to be very different. Neuroscience can provide information about the activation of a particular brain region, while clinical science can provide information about content (e.g., a depressotypic belief system). Both are important, and both can inform us about dimensions of vulnerability, but they provide very different types of knowledge. It is thus important to acknowledge that the chances that research will ever be able to map a one-to-one link between a brain structure, or a set of neural circuits, and a corresponding psychological variable appear to range from slim to none. Science fiction aside, we will never know the location of "meaning" in the brain, nor will we be able to translate the process of meaning making into a given set of neural circuits. With these differences and similarities in mind, we now turn to an examination of the antecedents, assumptions, and principles of the cognitive approach to behavior, and its clinical links, and to the antecedents, assumptions, and principles of cognitive neuroscience.

GUIDING ASSUMPTIONS OF COGNITIVE APPROACHES

A guiding assumption in the study of cognition is that the objective features of a stimulus are insufficient to predict human cognitive performance alone. Rather, mental functions play important mediating roles in determining a response to any particular stimulus. Put more simply, we do not all see objects, let alone more complex behavior, the same way. This is an elaboration of the basic stimulus–response model of behavior that includes mental operations as an intermediary step in the chain of events. These operations are what we find when we look inside the "black box" of the mind.

One approach by cognitive psychologists is to study the mental processes that produce reactions to stimuli and to identify the subcomponents that perform different mental operations on a stimulus that lead to a response. It is the combination of these elementary mental processes or operations that produce complex behavior (Posner & McLeod, 1982). To illustrate, consider the commonly accepted view that the time between a stimulus and a response is occupied by a series of processes or stages, some of which are mental operations, and many of which are arranged in such a fashion that one process does not begin until the preceding one has ended (Sternberg, 1969). Using this framework, researchers studying reaction time have developed methods in which the difference between average response times for two tasks is used to estimate the duration of the process by which they differ (Donders, 1868–1869/1969). This has enabled a more accurate study of mental operations and how they combine to produce complex performance. Understanding these basic mental operations thus forms the basis of the assumptions and principles that underlie the cognitive approach to human behavior, and as such may be informative about cognitive vulnerability to depression.

HISTORICAL AND CONTEMPORARY ISSUES

To fully appreciate contemporary developments in cognitive psychology it is important to consider the historical context from which they have arisen. Thus, prior to assessing contemporary aspects of the study of cognition, we address several important historical constructs and milestones in the study of cognition.

The dominance of behaviorism in the early decades of the 20th century temporarily impeded the development of methods for the study of the mind. The reemergence of interest in cognitive psychology has been traced by Anderson (1985) to developments in three areas. First, human factors research received a boost in World War II when practical information about human cognitive skills was in need to help improve responses to potentially lethal situations. The second development stemmed from advances in computer science, especially work that demonstrated the ability of computer programs to problem-solve. This work helped to establish the mind-as-computer metaphor that in some respects revolutionized thinking about cognition. Third, advances in the study of linguistics portrayed language acquisition and fluency as inherently complex abilities that could not be explained by behavioral theories. These forces pushed the agenda of cognitive psychology to the forefront of psychological science and helped to eclipse the previously dominant behavioral emphasis in these areas.

In many respects, the emergence of cognitive and information-processing approaches to emotional disorders can also be traced to a commitment by many scientists to integrate clinical and experimental psychological science. This is not the first time, however, that clinical interests looked explicitly to the ideas, concepts, and methods of basic psychological science. For example, the principles of learning theory developed in experimental laboratories in the 1930s (e.g., Guhtrie, 1935; Tolman, 1932) provided fertile ground for generating a diversity of applied and clinical research applications (Kanfer & Hagerman, 1985). These principles, of course, constituted the antecedents of clinical behaviorism, and once again, there are substantial benefits for theory, research, and clinical applications that draw upon work in the analysis of cognition.

Although it took a while to catch up, the influence of purely behavioral accounts of learning had a profound impact on clinical psychology. Theories of emotional disorder, which assumed the acquisition of maladaptive behavioral repertoires to be due to simplistic stimulus–response pairings, were challenged by a framework that admitted the possibility of cognitive mediation. This led to an interest in the role of thinking and reasoning in psychopathology. Bandura's (1969) influential work, for example, legitimized the study of cognitive variables such as expectancies, self-verbalizations, and predictions that had previously been excluded from accounts of human behavior and learning.

As the interest in cognitive accounts of disordered behavior grew, therapies were developed that capitalized on the idea that cognition might be an important clinical target. Although some of these ideas were straightforward extensions of behavioristic learning principles that went largely unverified (e.g., covert reinforcement; Cautela, 1970), at the very least this applied interest stimulated further attention to the clinical utility of cognitive constructs. Yet little in the way of any guiding paradigms with which to conceptualize the role and functioning of cognition in clinical problems was available; what existed instead was a broad area of interest and inquiry that recognized that maladaptive cognitions were part of emotional disorders (Ingram & Kendall, 1986).

Fortunately, from a conceptual standpoint, the growing recognition of the role of cognitive mediation in learning was soon accompanied by an influx of information from the neurosciences and computer sciences that focused the study of behavior change on questions of representation and constructive processes in perception (Pribram, 1986). Termed the *information-processing perspective*, clinical extensions of this viewpoint emphasized that humans are not merely passive recipients of information, but are instead active and selective seekers, creators, and users of information (Ingram & Kendall, 1986; Mahoney, 1990). Accounts of how people learn, which had previously only accepted stimuli, responses, and contingencies, started to consider deliberate cognitive activity as important; a wealth of meaningful activity occurring in the "black box" that behavioristic approaches had conceptually been unable to explore was now available for examination.

Attempts to define the basic principles of cognitive functioning, both in general and as they relate to clinical concerns, were made by a number of theorists. According to an early definition offered by Mahoney (1977), the basic tenets of a cognitive mediation perspective in clinical psychology were that (1) humans respond primarily to cognitive representations of the environment rather than to the environment per se; (2) these cognitive representations are related to the principles of learning; (3) most learning is cognitively mediated; and (4) thoughts, feelings, and behaviors influence one another.

The applied aspects of cognitive assumptions stemming from the recognition that thoughts, feelings, and behaviors influence each other can be seen in the premises of contemporary cognitive treatment approaches. More specifically, the assumption that thoughts, feelings, and behaviors influence each other leads to the postulates that (1) modifying cognition can lead to the corollary modification of maladaptive patterns of emotion and behavior, and (2) cognitive and behavioral change methods can be integrated for effective intervention concerning emotional distress. These assumptions have received support as evidenced by the data demonstrating the efficacy of a number of cognitive treatment approaches (see Hollon et al., 2006; Stewart & Chambless, 2009).

EVOLUTION FROM INFORMATION PROCESSING TO COGNITIVE NEUROSCIENCE

According to academic lore provided by the Cognitive Neuroscience Society (a academic society dedicated to mind and brain research), the term *cognitive neuroscience* was coined during a relatively casual conversation between the influential neuroscientist Michael Gazzaniga and the famous cognitive psychologist George Miller. These two researchers, as well as many other leaders in the fields of neuroscience and cognitive psychology, had been brought together for a dinner hosted by Rockefeller and Cornell Universities to discuss how the mind and brain work together. This conversation took place in the late 1970s at a time when the information-processing approach provided by the field of cognitive psychology could be readily melded with the growing repertoire of tools that were allowing neuroscientists to study intact healthy brains as they accomplished complex cognitive functions. Given this history, the field of cognitive neuroscience naturally overlaps with cognitive psychology, and in fact has its roots largely in cognitive psychophysiology. But whereas cognitive psychologists seek to understand the mind, researchers in cognitive neuroscience are concerned with understanding how these mental processes take place in the brain. The two areas influence each other on a continuous basis, since an understanding of mental structure can inform theories about brain functions and knowledge about neural mechanisms is useful in understanding mental structure.

Cognitive neuroscience is a study of how behavior and cognition are supported by the nervous system. Unlike most fields within the larger discipline of biological psychology, they will not always take a true reductionistic approach to the study of this relationship. Cognitive neuroscience tends to make the following assumptions: (1) behavior and cognition cause changes in physiology and (2) physiological changes can lead to changes in our behavior and cognition. But unlike their more reductionist colleagues, cognitive neuroscientists see physiological measures as a "window" into the mind. They are less likely to try to find the one-to-one map between physiology and cognition, at least not in their daily research. However, though they might not always act like reductionists (at a molecular level), their work generally reflects a philosophy of material monism.

Another important aspect of the general assumptions of the field of cognitive neuroscience is the belief that the brain, like cognition, must be seen as an interactive system made up of functionally divisible subprocessors. In this way, researchers in the domain of cognitive neuroscience can find a wealth of useful guidance and theoretical support via the direct study and integration of information-processing approaches and ideas of cognitive psychology. This is in part a reflection of the somewhat modularist notions that are adopted by many cognitive psychologists, which provide a blueprint for dissecting a complex cognitive process into separable, distinct, but yet interactive subprocesses that collectively result in some cognitive outcome. In both cognitive psychology and the field of cognitive neuroscience this tendency to pull apart a complex process in order to try to find the system's individual subcomponents has been adopted in order to avoid the dreaded "homunculus" problem.

In scientific philosophy the homunculus problem represents an unknowable agent within a system that plays a critical role in some function of interest, but is either too computationally complex or simply so poorly understood that the theory plagued by this shortfall is significantly hampered. A common example of the homunculus problem comes from the domain of vision theory. Imagine a person who is looking at a scene in the environment. The observer sees the objects in the environment as something separate from the self as if the images are being projected on the screen. A simple theory might propose that the light from the environment forms an image on the retina, much like a camera captures an image. Then something in the brain looks at these images, much like we would look at a still picture that the camera produced. This explanation of vision contains a homunculus because this theory does not provide an adequate explanation; all that has been done is to place a homunculus, or a little person, behind the eyes whose job it is to gaze at the retina. Therefore, the homunculus problem refers to any theoretical instance when there is a need for a "little man" to complete the theory. The philosopher Daniel Dennett (1991) has proposed the term "Cartesian theater" to characterize this kind of explanation for cognition.

Avoiding this homunculus problem is often accomplished by finding ways in which either the mind or the brain might break up these more complex processes into simpler and more tractable computational mechanisms that might be carried out by identifiable subprocessors or brain regions. This effort to situate the complex functions of the mind in separate components is consistent with many aspects of reductionism, which allows for the explanation of behavioral phenomena by analyzing them into separate parts, and then determining the properties and functions of these parts. Additionally, the goal is to understand the mind and brain as an interactive network, which is distributed over these many components, so that we can gain both from understanding each subsystem and by understanding how these subsystems are related and interconnected.

This notion of subdividing cognition or behavior fits very well with the historic biases and underpinnings of the field of cognitive neuroscience. Dating from as far back as the work of scientists such as Thomas Willis (1621–1675), Julien Jean-César Legallois (1770–1840), and François Magendie (1783–1840), we find the first discussions of physiological evidence of what would become known as the tenets of functional localization within the central nervous system. For example, Legallois discovered that if he were to lesion tissue in the medulla, this resulted in cessation of breathing, thus leading to an understanding that medullar function supports respiration. This discovery is thought to be the first direct evidence of localization of function within the brain (Finger, 1994).

This exploration of the direct connection between anatomical structure and behavioral function was continued by researchers such as Franz Joseph Gall (1785–1828) and Johann Spurzheim (1776–1832) via the development of the phrenological tradition. *Phrenology* refers to the study of the topography of the skull as a way to measure individual differences in personality, cognitive function, and other aspects of a person's character. Gall himself was said to have identified and localized 27 individual trails including functions such as pride and an instinct for self-defense. Despite the fact the phrenology is not held in high regard, in part because it was used to buttress a kind of "scientifically" supported racism, and also because the empirical methods employed by its supporters were a perfect example of pseudoscience, nonetheless, one core assumption that underlies phrenology, the idea that basic cognitive faculties are localized to distinct "organs" within the brain, represents a kind of building block for the development of modern cognitive neuroscience.

Furthermore, this idea of functional distinctions could then be combined with research such as the landmark work of Korbinian Brodmann (1868–1918) who was able to structurally distinguish between cortical regions via the study of cytoarchitecture, or the study of the differences in neuronal shape, size, and organization that exist between areas of brain tissue. Brodmann's primary tools for his work were cellular staining techniques that had been recently developed by scientists such as Camillo Golgi (1843–1926) and Franz Nissl (1860–1919). These staining methods allowed Brodmann, and the researchers who continued his work, to visualize neuron cell bodies and thus draw quite precise boundaries between individual regions of cortical tissue. Brodmann hypothesized that the different cytoarchitectural regions that he was identifying would prove to have very distinct functions. This hypothesis has been soundly supported by the intervening 100 years of research. The outcome of all this work has been a somewhat imprecise but ever-developing understanding of the functional architecture of the human brain.

NEUROSCIENCE MODELS OF EMOTION

When Plato (429–347 BCE) and Aristotle (384–322 BCE) divided the functions of the human mind via a tripartite model (intellect, emotion/desire, and cognition), they effectively argued that cognition and emotion are distinct and nonoverlapping domains of human behavior. In fact they argued that intellect and desire were in direct conflict. This division between the study of emotion and the study of cognition has a long history and was maintained, in all but exceptional cases, throughout much of the history of psychology. In what follows, we discuss these exceptional cases as well as the researchers who have argued that it is useful to consider emotion when trying to understand cognition more generally.

In a text edited by Lane and Nadel (2000), titled *Cognitive Neuroscience of Emotion*, the editors provide a nice overview of why it is possible and likely advantageous to apply cognitive neuroscience perspectives to the understanding of emotion. The arguments include the idea that emotions in many ways direct or provide awareness of ongoing cognition, that cognition and emotion involve many overlapping behavioral and neurophysiological systems, and that some of the most fruitful ways to study emotion are via cognitive neuroscience methods (Lane, Nadel, Allen, & Kaszniak, 2000). These arguments apply when discussing our general understanding of emotion and, we would argue, that they also apply when we consider the more specific domain of depression vulnerability.

The growing acceptance of emotion as a theoretical area of inquiry in the cognitive neurosciences has lead to another potentially fruitful and relevant avenue of questions, specifically questions regarding the role that emotion might play evolutionarily. Hence, we note the role evolution might play in selecting for different patterns of emotional response, a question that seems of direct relevance to the question of why a disordered syndrome such as depression might continue to emerge in our species.

Additionally, the next section reviews two dominant classes of cognitive neuroscience models of emotion. For someone new to this domain, the distinctions between these two kinds of models may seem subtle, but these two models and the resulting research designed to either choose between them or find common ground has influenced much of the cognitive neuroscience research on emotion in the last 40 years. Borod (2000) provides a nice overview of the history of this debate when she discusses the theoretical debate that happened in the early 1980s between Robert Zajonc (1980, 1984) and Richard Lazarus (1982, 1984). Zajonc argued that emotion precedes cognition and is not part of our cognitive processing system (consistent with the historic models discussed above). Lazarus argued for the opposite timeline, that is, cognition precedes emotion. Below we review models that fall into these two general camps.

Physiological–Somatic Models of Emotion

The Zajonc-like category of emotion theory hypothesizes that emotion processing is activated upon the perception of a stimulus that has emotional significance in our environment, as in the case of seeing a face (Tracy & Robins, 2008). This stimulus elicits a particular bodily response or physiological reaction that is very directly related to the nature of that emotional stimulus (Lange & James, 1922). Following this physiological response, the experience of emotion emerges as a direct result of the driving physiological state. One of the first examples of this class of theories was independently developed by Carl Lange (1887) and William James (1884), who noted:

> Our natural way of thinking about these standard emotions is that the mental perception of some fact excites the mental affection called the emotion, and that this latter state of mind gives rise to the bodily expression. My thesis on the contrary is that the bodily changes follow directly the perception of the exciting fact, and that our feeling of the same changes as they occur is the emotion. Common sense says, we lose our fortune, are sorry and weep; we meet a bear, are frightened and run; we are insulted by a rival, are angry and strike. The hypothesis here to be defended says that this order of sequence is incorrect, that the one mental state is not immediately induced by the other, that the bodily manifestations must first be interposed between, and that the more rational statement is that we feel sorry because we cry, angry because we strike, afraid because we tremble, and not that we cry, strike, or tremble, because we are sorry, angry, or fearful, as the case may be. (p. 190)

Despite the very early beginning of this kind of theory, many researchers are elaborating upon the James–Lange theory of emotion by investigating the interaction between the physiological responses such as those generated in the autonomic nervous system and the experience of emotion. For example, Damasio and colleagues consider emotion to be an unconscious physiological system that activates when an evolutionarily significant stimulus is presented (Damasio, 1998; Damasio et al., 2000). This model by Damasio and others is generally referred to as the somatic marker theory. This theory argues that there is a brain–body feedback loop, a system that takes into account the idea that emotion is not merely the conscious perception of the physiological change that is taking place but is also influenced by unconscious feedback from the body that is essential to emotional perception. Evidence for the unconscious, bioregulatory nature of emotion presented by Damasio et al. (2000) suggests that feeling an emotion draws upon both cortical and subcortical structures that belong to patterns of neural activity that have developed throughout the evolution of our species. These researchers posit that emotion be considered a whole-body regulation mechanism closely related to maintaining homeostasis, as feeling an emotion draws upon brain structures that both receive internal signals, via the peripheral nervous system, and distribute these signals, via the spinal cord. Considering basic emotion processes as related to homeostasis is important for the theory that has driven much of the work done by Damasio and colleagues. Damasio's somatic marker hypothesis considers the regulatory nature of emotion as an example of how integrative emotion systems affect more than conscious perception, as in cases of how stress can lead to fatigue and heart disease.

The theoretical construct of *motivated attention* has also generally characterized the function of emotion as serving a somewhat reflexive, unconscious role. The function of emotion, according to this theory, is that it provides an individual organism with some particular action set, whether of an approach type or of an avoidance type, that is the most appropriate way to act given the presence of an emotional stimulus (Bradley et al., 2001, 2003; Frijda, 1986; Lang, 1984). This theory states that evolutionarily significant stimuli in our environment activate the subcortical arousal networks necessary for action sets to be applied (Cuthbert et al., 2003; Lane et al., 1997). Bradley and colleagues have put forth distinct sets of stimuli that allow motivated attention to be tested. Among their methodological tools, the International Affective Picture System (IAPS; Lang, Bradley, & Cuthbert, 1999) has been shown to be an efficient tool used to stimulate appetitive or defensive responses significant to the evolutionary mechanisms regarded as emotion. The theory behind this method of emotion elicitation is that salient pictures containing emotionally significant material will activate the same neural circuitry related to appetitive and defensive action that is required to assess stimuli in our natural environment (Bradley et al., 2001). In this research, it is assumed that the semantic content of the pictures (i.e., the situation depicted) elicits a physiological response comparable to encountering the real-life event. Work by Lang, Bradley, and colleagues has also provided a good deal of insight into the methodological tools that can be used to measure emotion. In a very nice review, for example, Bradley and Lang (2000) provide a overview of both the response systems that can be measured and the appropriate tools for collecting the "data of emotion" (p. 244).

An additional theory that should be considered by any researcher interested in the neuropsychology of emotion was developed by Öhman and colleagues (Öhman, 1987, 1999; Öhman, Flykt, & Lundqvist, 2000). Öhman's theory also sees these unconscious mechanisms of emotion as serving an evolutionary purpose. Specifically, Öhman argues that emotion works via an evolutionarily programmed attentional bias that helps our attentional system to automatically capture emotion stimuli that may not be captured by our cognitively controlled, goal-driven selective attention system. This kind of automatic shift of attention to emotionally threatening stimuli is then paired with automatic physiological responses, such as via the autonomic nervous system. Thus, as with the other models discussed above, the emotional responses that work via unconscious physiological response systems are going to have their effect and change human behavior without the need for cognitively demanding processes such as controlled selective attention being brought online.

Two-Factor Models of Emotion

While researchers such as William James, Arne Öhman, and Antonio Damasio draw our attention to how emotion can function at an unconscious level and via primarily physiological response systems, other researchers, such as Lazarus (1982, 1984), have argued that cognitive processes such as attention or memory play a critical role in the initial experience of emotion. The theories based on underlying, unconscious mechanisms of emotion are important for understanding behavior, but in order to present an extensive discussion of the nature of emotion, we will likely benefit from also considering the role played by cognition. As an alternative to a James–Lange-like theory of emotion, one of the first two-factor theories was developed by Stanley Schachter and Jerome Singer (1962). The two-factor theory essentially argues that the influence of both physiological arousal and cognitive functions are combined to generate an emotional experience.

One important thing to understand about these models that combine physiology and cognition, which we typically refer to as two-factor models, is that these models necessarily do not deny the role played by physiological responses in determining emotion perception or the nature of emotional experience. The models that fall into this category instead ask questions about how, when, and where in the brain is the emotion network functioning. Some influential research that has discussed this very integrative approach to emotion processing comes from the work of Tucker (Derryberry & Tucker, 1992; Tucker, 1981; Tucker & Williamson, 1984). A second important researcher contributing to the development of more subcortically oriented two-factor models is LeDoux (LeDoux, 1998, 2000). Both Tucker and LeDoux provide a clear discussion of how cortical and subcortical structures like the amygdala and neocortical structures work in concert to allow for the many behavioral consequences of emotion processing of such things as subjective experience, motivation, and stimulus evaluation.

Providing a good example of this kind of model, Derryberry and Tucker (1992) offer a very thorough review of the neuroanatomical mechanisms of emotion. In much the same way that the consideration of evolutionary mechanisms has influenced more somatic models, likewise researchers like Tucker have also employed an evolutionary framework. Tucker argues that more primitive brainstem structures regulate the physiological emotion responses of the body and thus support the instrumental functions of emotion. Later in our evolutionary history structures that now make up our limbic system developed to provide sensitivity to a wider range of emotion-related stimuli and more plasticity in our response mechanisms. After this cortical brain region began to evolve, these structures allowed for even more fine-grain differentiation between emotion-related representations and the recruitment of cognitive processes that aid in control mechanisms, learning, and elaborative or interpretive processes. Applying evidence from functional neuroimaging techniques to support this phylogenetic argument, Derryberry and Tucker (1992) speculate that the subcortical structures specific to the initial processing of emotion have developed directly from more primitive structures that perform basic regulatory, motor, and arousal functions. These emotional structures, including the hypothalamus and the limbic system, are organized so that appraisal and judgment can be most efficient. Furthermore, Derryberry and Tucker discuss structures within the hippocampus that play a large role in emotion processing through the application of information in long-term memory stores to emotional assessment, anticipation, and planning.

Relevant to the topics in the current volume, the issue of individual differences has been commonly addressed by multiple two-factor models of emotion. Cortical structures and, in particular, the lateralization of cerebral hemisphere activation, has been argued to be an important differentiating parameter between individuals who process emotional information differently. In a review of his work on laterality, Davidson (2003) considers the effects of emotion on language processing using evidence from brain imaging and electrophysiological techniques. His work has found that the efficiency of eliciting an emotional reaction from participants in his lab is influenced by individual differences in emotion processing (Davidson, 2003). His elicitation measures, such as watching an emotional film or viewing emotional imagery, are used as a means of identifying the underlying patterns of individual biases in attention and susceptibility to the content of an emotional stimulus (Davidson, 2003; Davidson et al., 1990; Wheeler, Davidson, & Tomarken, 1993). Unique circumstances arise when dealing with emotionality and personal experience. Davidson's term "affective style" refers to a reaction that is unique to each participant as a result of his or her adaptation to the environment and the individual's ability to regulate emotion (Davidson, 1994, 2003; Davidson, Putnam, & Larson, 2000). Davidson speculates that the differences in how we process emotional information individually are influenced by the amygdala and activity in the prefrontal cortex, a brain region assumed to play an important role in higher order cognition (Davidson, 2001, 2002; Wheeler, 1993).

Anticipation and inhibition are important roles undertaken by subcortical structures, but specific areas located within the prefrontal cortex are also involved in these cognitive functions (Davidson, 2001, 2002; Wheeler, 1993). Davidson's claim is that a specific hemisphere of the prefrontal cortex is activated under circumstances that involve decisions about whether to approach or withdraw from a particular object or behavior, and lateral activation is especially necessary when goals are inconsistent with the initial information appraised from a stimulus, such as when pain from an injury is encountered while eating a delicious fruit or potential food can be made of a dangerous animal (Davidson, 2003; Davidson et al., 2000). The prefrontal cortex influences reactions when faced with uncertainty or when a novel response is necessary for more elaborate goals (Davidson, 2003). Davidson focuses on individual biases in emotion responses localized in the prefrontal cortex and how hemispheric specificity can influence these particular reactions.

Davidson has found more activation in a particular hemisphere relevant to the valence of emotional stimuli. His laterality hypothesis has successfully predicted whether individuals will respond with a valence bias, as in when stronger activation for negative information is observed among certain individuals. Much of Davidson's work shows a laterality bias for positive stimuli in the left hemisphere, while the right hemisphere seems to be activated by negative material. Davidson has attributed each hemisphere with its respective valence-processing bias. There is a considerable amount of literature documenting hemispheric differences in prefrontal cortex activity as a function of emotional valence (Davidson, 1992, 2003; Heller, 1993).

Subcortical anatomy is also considered by Davidson (2001, 2002, 2003) as he illustrates the importance of the amygdala and its crucial function in the motivation of further processing so that attentional resources can be directed in proportion to the emotional significance of a stimulus. Davidson assumes a general role of the amygdala in emotion processing, though his evidence suggests a negativity bias in this structure that is reasonably due to an evolutionary proclivity to react aversively when confronted with novel stimuli as a defensive precaution (Davidson, 2003). After initial assessment of an environmental stimulus and the immediate reactions necessary are considered, a more complete evaluation can make sense of ambiguous properties. Therefore, Davidson's position regards cortical processing as playing a larger role in evaluating emotional stimuli, as emotional information requires more advanced processing than that which can occur at the arousal level in subcortical structure, all this being consistent with a two-factor model (Davidson, 2003). This characterization is based in part on neurological patient data, such as a sample of 160 lesion patients examined by Gainotti (1972), who found catastrophic or anxious–depressive reactions more frequently among patients with damage to the left frontal cortex and euphoric/indifference reactions among patients with right frontal damage. A large number of corroborative studies have also employed resting EEG measures as a way of examining both prefrontal cortex asymmetries (see Davidson, 2003, for a review).

A theoretical framework that adds to the prefrontal cortex valence theories of Davidson is a second theory of hemispheric lateralization for emotion sometimes referred to as the "circumplex model of emotion" (Heller & Nitschke, 1997; Heller, Nitschke, & Miller, 1998). This model postulates that the posterior right hemisphere is responsible for all perception of emotion, regardless of valence, while the anterior frontal regions are differentially mediated in accordance with the Davidson-like valence model for the experience of emotion (Adolphs, Damasio, Tranel, & Damasio, 1996; Heller, 1993; Heller & Nitschke, 1997). Researchers arguing for this model have also emphasized the need to understand more stable patterns of emotion processing, such as variance seen across people with different personality styles (such as extraversion or impulsivity) and across different patient populations (such as individuals with anxiety or depression). According to the circumplex model, multiple aspects of cognition play a central role in emotion, not just the internal experience of mood or emotion, controlled by frontal lobe regions, as studies by researchers like Davidson suggest. The circumplex model also focuses on the role that posterior right hemisphere regions of the cortex play in a person's evaluation of external emotional stimuli such as faces or prosodic emotional cues in the voice (Borod, 1993; Heller, 1997).

SUMMARY

In this chapter, we noted that the field of cognitive psychology approaches the understanding of both behavior and emotion from the perspective that objective features of a stimulus are insufficient to predict human cognition and behavior alone. Rather, mental functions play important mediating roles in determining a response to any particular stimulus. This is an elaboration of the basic stimulus–response model of behavior that includes cognitive operations as an intermediary step in the chain of events. Cognitive neuroscience contributes to this hypothesized causal chain by adding the assumptions that behavior and cognition also cause changes in physiology and/or physiological changes can lead to changes in our behavior and cognition. Additionally, a general assumption of cognitive psychology and cognitive neuroscience is the belief that both the workings of cognition and the workings of the brain must be seen as interactive systems made up of functionally divisible subprocessors. In this way, researchers in these domains can find a wealth of useful guidance and theoretical support via the direct study and integration of information-processing approaches and the corresponding working model of functional localization in brain processes that guides much of the cognitive neuroscience research.

Turning more specifically to the domain of cognitive and cognitive neuroscience models that try to understand emotional functions, we noted the long philosophical tradition dating back to Plato and Aristotle that divides the functions of emotion and cognition into distinct categories. We also noted, however, that unlike the early Greeks, contemporary cognitive and cognitive neuroscience theorists argue about the degree to which cognition and emotion are distinct systems. There is a clear consensus that even if these domains of human behavior are functionally or anatomically distinct, they are clearly interactive systems that "collaborate" in their production of human behavior. As we discussed, one way to organize the broader theoretical discussion about how emotions influence behavior, and how they are instantiated in the mind and brain is to talk about two classes of emotion models generally referred to as the physiological–somatic models of emotion and the two-factor models of emotion. As we discussed, the physiological–somatic models generally argue that emotion processing is activated upon the perception of a stimulus that has emotional significance in our environment, and that this stimulus elicits a particular bodily response or physiological reaction that emerges during the experience of emotion. The other major perspective we examined was the two-factor idea, which argues that the influence of both physiological arousal and cognitive functions are combined to generate an emotional experience.

4

Methodological Strategies and Issues in the Study of Vulnerability to Depression

Before we examine the research illustrating the role of cognitive and neuroscience variables in depression risk, we examine the strategies and methods used to generate this research. We start with an examination of the concepts of distal and proximal vulnerability, and then discuss and critique the methods that have been used to investigate these types of risk. We also examine basic methodological strategies that underlie cognitive neuroscience research on depression risk. Because our goal is to examine issues that are of particular relevance to vulnerability research, we will not highlight general methodological considerations in the conduct of research (e.g., the need for control groups, experimenter bias, demand characteristics). These basic considerations are critical for producing meaningful research, but are beyond the scope of the present volume. Readers who are interested in research design issues as they apply to clinical research in general or to depression research in particular are referred to several outstanding sources (e.g., Haaga & Solomon, 1993; Kazdin, 2003; Kendall et al., 1987; Kendall & Butcher, 1982; Roberts & Ilardi, 2003; Sher & Trull, 1996; Smith & Rhodewalt, 1991).

DISTAL AND PROXIMAL VULNERABILITY

As we noted in Chapter 2, risk variables must be present before the onset of a depressive episode. As such, risk can be either distal or proximal in nature. *Proximal risk* reflects variables that precede depression onset, but do so close in time to the onset of the disorder. For example, the occurrence of a negative life event that triggers a depressive response that turns into a diagnosable (after 2 weeks) major depressive disorder would be a proximal variable. In contrast, *distal factors* are also present before onset but, at least relative to proximal variables, occur temporally farther from the appearance of depression. Hence, if a negative life event occurs that triggers a physiological process that eventually leads to depression, this event would be seen as a more distal cause in comparison to the physiological process. Or from a cognitive perspective, the occurrence of an event might lead to an attribution on which the individual blames him- or herself. If this attribution then leads to a biological process that eventuates in a depressive episode, the attribution can be seen as a more distal variable.

The distinction between proximal and distal vulnerability is relative in most cases. That is, if variable *B* in the causal chain occurs temporally farther from onset than variable *A*, then *B* is the distal variable. However, if variable *C* occurs even farther from the onset than *B*, *A* remains proximal, *C* is distal, and *B* becomes either "less" distal or "more" proximal. The possible permutations are theoretically endless, but in practice there are fewer possibilities.

It is important to recognize that, although the distinction between proximal and distal vulnerability is recognized by many models, different models draw the line between these variables in different places. For instance, Figure 4.1 represents distal and proximal factors in Beck's (1967, 1987) theory as interpreted by Abramson, Alloy, and Metalsky (1988). In this case of a "short" time line, the presence of a negative self-schema is seen as a distal variable, while cognitive distortions and a negative cognitive triad are seen as proximal causes of depressive symp-

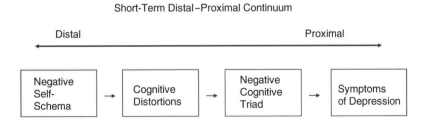

FIGURE 4.1. Short-term depiction of distal and proximal factors.

toms. Both contribute to the development of depression but do so at different points in time.

Distal and proximal constructs can, however, also be conceptualized on a much more long-term continuum. For example, consider an understanding of risk factors that is extended to the developmental antecedents of vulnerability (e.g., Abela & Hankin, 2008), as illustrated in Figure 4.2. According to this view, developmental antecedents reflect very distal vulnerability factors because they occur considerably before the appearance of a depressive disorder. However, the negative self-schema construct remains a distal feature relative to the negative cognitive triad, but now becomes a more proximal factor in relationship to developmentally rooted variables.

Distal and Proximal Causes of Onset and Maintenance

It is important to note that conceptual differences between distal and proximal factors is not limited to the onset of the disorder. Distal and proximal factors can also be distinguished by the role they play in the perpetuation of depression. Hence, researchers can search for the variables that place individuals at risk for an extended case of depression. As an example, several models have explicitly suggested that ruminative cognitive processes serve to maintain depression (Ingram, 1984; Nolen-Hoeksema, 1991; Pyszczynski & Greenberg, 1987; Teasdale, 1983, 1988; Watkins, Moberly, & Moulds, 2008). Active rumination during a depressed state would be considered a proximal cause of the perpetua-

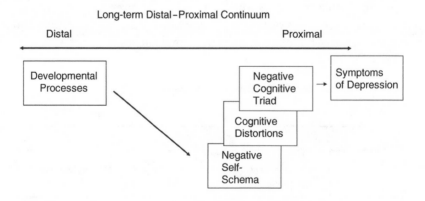

FIGURE 4.2. Longer-term depiction of distal and proximal factors.

tion of depression, but those factors that predispose people to ruminate in response to negative mood states could be considered distal.

METHODOLOGICAL STRATEGIES AND ISSUES IN THE STUDY OF PROXIMAL VULNERABILITY

To examine the methodological foundations of data on vulnerability, and to provide a context for our subsequent review of vulnerability data, we discuss here several established research strategies. We start with a discussion of methodological strategies for the examination of proximal vulnerability. Although there are any number of research designs that could be brought to bear on the study of vulnerability-related phenomena, here we concentrate on several of the major designs that have been used to study proximal vulnerability, and examine their strengths and limitations in the study of vulnerability. Specifically, we examine (1) cross-sectional designs, (2) remission designs, and (3) priming designs. Although we discuss these as separate strategies, it is important to note that, depending upon the questions of particular research interest, considerable overlap among these designs can be found in the literature.

Cross-Sectional Designs in Proximal Vulnerability Research

The general methodological strategy underlying cross-sectional designs follows the established research tradition of dividing research participants into groups according to individual difference variables and then examining differences between these groups on some other variable of interest. In depression research, this typically means selecting a group of depressed individuals and then comparing them to a control group of nondepressed subjects.

Advantages and Limitations

Cross-sectional designs have generated a considerable amount of data on the factors that characterize depression (Haaga, Dyck, & Ernst, 1991; Scher, Ingram, & Segal, 2005), and are invaluable as a tool for describing the features of depression. Such descriptive efforts can also provide potentially important clues for researchers seeking to understand the causal features of depression. As such, cross-sectional studies have generated a considerable body of data. However, the limitations of cross-sectional studies for understanding vulnerability are considerable.

Limitations stem from several basic considerations. The first concerns the type of theoretical model the investigator seeks to examine. Consider the cognitive model proposed by Beck as an example. By definition, the vulnerability factors that can be derived from such models are cognitive in nature. If, however, it is the case that only a subset of depressed people are depressed for cognitive reasons, as suggested by Abramson and Alloy (Abramson et al., 1988; Abramson & Alloy, 1990; Abramson, Metalsky, & Alloy, 1989; Alloy, Hartlage, & Abramson, 1988), then cross-sectionally comparing individuals who are selected only on the basis of being depressed is an inappropriate test of a cognitive model; individuals selected may be depressed for a variety of reasons, some of which have little to do with cognitive factors. Thus, there is likely to be too much error variance in such a sample to conduct any meaningful test of cognitive hypotheses, particularly if the proportion of individuals with noncognitive depression is relatively large in these studies. Although we have used cognitive models to illustrate this limitation, this concern applies to any design that employs depression as the basis for group comparisons.

A second and more fundamental limitation of cross-sectional studies concerns how data pertain to the causes of depression. In particular, cross-sectional designs are explicitly correlational in nature and do not allow for a differentiation between causal variables, consequential variables, or third variable causality (Garber & Hollon, 1991). Thus, although research has established a fairly clear picture of the functioning of various processes *in* a depressed state, these processes do not necessarily apply to the onset or perpetuation of depression. To infer causality we must demonstrate temporal antecedence: the feature must precede the onset of the disorder (Garber & Hollon, 1991), which correlational studies such as cross-sectional approaches cannot provide.

Are Causal Inferences Possible from Cross-Sectional Designs?

Causal inferences about the onset of depression are difficult to accurately make from cross-sectional designs. Nevertheless, there can be value in understanding causation in the data generated from cross-sectional designs. Causality is not synonymous with onset, although it tends to be treated that way. Given that cross-sectional designs assess individuals when they are in the midst of a depressive episode, one that is presumably being maintained by some set of factors, such studies may be relevant for understanding the factors that are causally linked to the *perpetuation* of depression (recall from our discussion in Chapter 1 that depression can last, by some estimates, up to 2 years). The features assessed in the depressed state by cross-sectional designs may therefore have a considerable degree of relevance for vulnerability if we keep in mind the broader perspective that views causality across a wide spectrum. Cross-sectional designs can thus be appropriate to assess vulnerability if the focus of these designs is on vulnerability to the perpetuation of the depressed state. It is important to note, however, that it is incumbent on researchers employing a cross-sectional design to specify how the variables studied may pertain to vulnerability to the perpetuation of depression.

Remission Designs

Some remission studies represent a category of cross-sectional designs. Rather than studying individuals currently in a depressed state, however, these designs examine individuals who were once, but who are no longer, depressed (i.e., in remission).[1] Participants can be identified either through longitudinal analyses, where they are followed from the depressed state to the nondepressed state (e.g., Segal et al., 2006), or retrospectively, where individuals are identified who at some point in the past had a depressive disorder (Gemar, Segal, Sagrati, & Kennedy, 2001; Ingram, Bernet, & McLaughlin, 1994; Miranda & Persons, 1988). Additionally, while it is necessary that research participants have previously experienced depression, it is wise to exclude them if they have also experienced other psychopathological states (e.g., a psychotic disorder). This rule-out parallels the methodological practice of many cross-sectional studies that exclude the occurrence of many other DSM-defined disorders (e.g., bipolar disorder, substance abuse disorder, psychotic disorder). As with cross-sectional studies as a whole, designs of this type can evaluate existing differences between formerly depressed and nondepressed individuals in a descriptive psychopathology fashion, or they can introduce some theory-specified event and then examine subsequent reactions.

---

[1]These studies can include participants who are in remission or who have recovered. There are important distinctions between these concepts, but because these tend to be described as remission studies in the literature, we follow this convention even if a particular study might have examined recovered rather than remitted individuals.

Advantages and Limitations

Owing to their conceptual overlap, cross-sectional and remission studies share very similar advantages. For example, remission studies can be helpful for understanding the longer term functioning of depressed individuals in a way that purely cross-sectional studies cannot. Unfortunately, remission designs in and of themselves may not be able to achieve their aims of assessing the presence of risk factors; these data may provide information about the stability of some factors, but only if there is theoretical or empirical reason to believe that the factors assessed are not only stable but are also continuously empirically accessible after remission.

The limitations of remission designs then reside, much as with purely cross-sectional designs, not in the design itself, but rather in how data generated from the design are interpreted, specifically the acceptance of null hypotheses. If we examine the cognitive literature, for instance, in a number of published reports researchers have been unable to detect evidence of dysfunctional cognitive factors once depression has remitted (Dobson & Shaw, 1986, 1987; Fennell & Campbell, 1984; Hamilton & Abramson, 1983; Persons & Rao, 1985; Segal & Dobson, 1992), leading to the interpretation that cognitive factors cannot be causal but are instead consequences or concomitants of the depression (Barnett & Gotlib, 1988). However, as with any design, null results can be obtained for a variety of reasons, making it difficult to disentangle whether the hypothesis is not true or whether other factors are obscuring the ability of the design to detect supportive evidence.

In the case of many remission studies, the failure to distinguish between accessibility and availability suggests that null results may be obtained because these studies have not adequately modeled the complexity of diathesis–stress models (Hollon, 1992). For example, in the cognitive arena, rather than viewing depressive schemas as structures that are static, even the earliest cognitive depression models (Beck, 1963, 1967) posited that individuals vulnerable to depression possess maladaptive schemas that are dormant *until activated* in response to stressful life events (Beck, 1987; Ingram, 1984; Teasdale, 1983, 1988). Segal and Shaw (1986) nicely articulate this view by emphasizing the idea that cognitive diathesis–stress approaches view stressful events as activating a "latent but reactive" schema that provides access to an elaborate system of negative content. Once activated, a pattern of negative self-referent information processing that leads to depression is initiated. This is the essence of a diathesis–stress approach to depression and corresponding cognitive vulnerability. Thus, given such a conceptualization, to have causal significance it is neither empirically nor theoretically necessary to require that variables that are salient during a depressive episode persist and be equally salient after the episode has ended.

Priming Designs

In line with diathesis–stress conceptualizations, a number of psychopathology variables are assumed to be discernible only within the context of eliciting stimuli that challenge the homeostasis of the individual (Segal & Ingram, 1994). As Hollon (1992) has noted, for instance, research investigating biological systems thought to be linked to affective disorders has established that dysregulation in these systems is apparent only following psychological or pharmacological challenges and not under ordinary circumstances (e.g., Depue & Iacono, 1989; Depue et al., 1985).

Most diathesis–stress perspectives thus necessitate that triggering agents be incorporated into evaluations of the vulnerability (for an exception, however, see the description of the Temple–Wisconsin Project in Chapter 5). Hence, in order to understand vulnerability, the logic underlying priming studies is to incorporate activation processes (represented as stress in diathesis–stress models) in combination with proposed diatheses (e.g., negative self-referent cognitive structures) (see Scher et al., 2005, and Segal & Ingram, 1994, for reviews). Only relatively recently, however, have psychological studies of depression, by virtue of relying on priming assumptions, begun to methodologically model the complexity of the theoretical proposals they seek to test (Hollon, 1992).

Modeling Stress: Types of Activation

A variety of theoretical approaches specify factors that can serve as activating agents. For example, several researchers have suggested a link between self-focused attention and depression (see Ingram, 1990; Pyszczynski & Greenberg, 1987) and, in fact, data have suggested that increased levels of self-focused attention are a risk factor for negative affect (Ingram et al., 1988; Ingram, Johnson, Bernet, Dombeck, & Rowe, 1992). It would thus be theoretically reasonable to induce self-focus in vulnerable people and then determine whether depressotypic processing ensues.

Despite the availability of a variety of different primes, studies have typically employed mood as the prime, with the underlying assumption that affective and cognitive processes are reciprocal and closely intertwined. Hence, cognition and affect are assumed to be intricately embedded within associative webs so that each affects the other, but in cognitive models cognition is treated as "first among equals" (Haaga et al., 1991). Mood-priming studies thus derive from, and represent logical tests of, existing models.

Regardless of the type of activating event that is employed, we believe that it is important for investigators to specify the assumptions as to what processes a priming process is affecting. In cognitive priming work, for example, studies that use mood inductions usually assume that mood serves as a direct activating agent. Additionally, the parameters of the activating stimuli may vary in their specificity. For instance, some theoretical assumptions may be so general that no specific type of activating events need be specified; biological challenge models do not necessarily rely on stresses that are specific to a particular theory or paradigm, but instead tend to focus on "generic" stresses to study the activation of dysregulation (e.g., exposing research participants to math problems; Depue & Kleiman, 1979).

Regardless of the type of priming induction, data must demonstrate either changes on the variables specified to be a function of the prime (e.g., pre- and postdifferences), or alternatively differences between randomly assigned primed versus nonprimed groups. This is the basic logic underlying classic experimental manipulation checks. It is also important to emphasize that these states must be assessed independently of the activation processes that they are presumed to effect; if a mood prime is used, then measures are needed to empirically verify that mood has been affected. Likewise, studies seeking to manipulate, for example, self-focused attention need to demonstrate that this state was in fact induced (Ingram, 1991).

If control groups are used in a between-subjects design, both groups must also show priming effects; otherwise, data are inherently confounded. For example, if a mood-priming procedure is used, remitted and never depressed individuals should show similar levels of sad mood after the induction. If only one group (e.g., formerly depressed individuals) experiences sad mood, or significantly greater sad mood, it is impossible to disentangle subsequent differences; are differences attributable to the presence of now detectable risk variables, or to the fact that vulnerable but not vulnerable individuals feel bad (or are self-focused, or have experienced expressed emotion, etc.)?

Advantages and Limitations

The obvious advantage of priming designs is that they more closely model the complexities of the diathesis–stress assumptions. Priming designs thus enable the study of hypothetically key variables when symptoms are not currently present, allowing a distinction to be made between processes that are symptomatic of depression and those that may precede and thus pose risk for depression. As such, they represent a powerful way to begin to test the proximal aspects of vulnerability to depression.

One limitation that is commonly noted for priming designs is the scar hypothesis. As first proposed by Lewinsohn, Steinmetz, Larson, and Franklin (1981), the scar hypothesis suggests that observed deficits in depression may represent an effect, or a scar, of the disorder rather than a cause, particularly a cause of an initial onset. Although intriguing, this hypothesis has received little empirical support (e.g., Beevers, Rhode, Stice, & Nolen-Hoeksema, 2007; Shea, Leon, Mueller, & Solomon, 1996). Another limitation serves more as a cautionary note rather than as a limitation of priming designs per se. That is, the demonstration that a theory-specific variable becomes emergent in a priming study is not evidence that that variable in fact plays a causal role. Research must demonstrate that such variables are in fact associated with the return of depression. In fact, two studies reported by Segal (Segal, Gemar, & Williams, 1999; Segal et al., 2006) have shown that primed variables can predict the recurrence of depression 2 years after treatment, although these data cannot speak to vulnerability to the initial episode.

METHODOLOGICAL STRATEGIES AND ISSUES IN THE STUDY OF DISTAL VULNERABILITY

Having examined research strategies for investigating vulnerability from a proximal perspective, we turn now to methodological issues and research strategies that are relevant to the assessment of the distal components of vulnerability. Our particular focus on distal variables tends toward vulnerability patterns that are developed early in life. As such, these early patterns may reflect the developmentally determined antecedents of adult depression. Accordingly, many (although not all) research paradigms relevant to distal vulnerability focus on the examination of vulnerability factors in childhood.

We begin by examining high-risk designs, which can be divided into the more common high-risk offspring design and the quite uncommon high-risk parental design. We then examine various longitudinal approaches and cross-sequential designs and conclude with a discussion of retrospective designs, and a subcategory of these designs, experimental retrospective strategies.

High-Risk Offspring Designs

As we noted in Chapter 2, many of the first investigations of vulnerability to psychopathology, specifically, vulnerability to schizophrenia, assessed the offspring of individuals with a disorder. The early studies by Mednick and Schulsinger (1968) and Kety et al. (1968) investigating the offspring of Danish schizophrenic mothers established this strategy as a way to help understand the transmission of risk factors, and hence a number of early schizophrenia vulnerability studies employed this approach (e.g., the Stony Brook High-Risk Study—Weintraub, 1987; the Minnesota High-Risk Study—Rolf, 1972; Garmezy & Devine, 1984; the St. Louis High-Risk Study—Worland, Janes, Anthony, McGinnis, & Cass, 1984).

A critical assumption underlying this approach is that children are at increased risk for developing a disorder similar to that of one or both of their parents. Hence, the offspring of depressed parents should possess the factors that place them at risk for depression, and indeed data suggest that the children of depressed mothers are six times more likely to develop depression than the children of nondepressed mothers (see Goodman & Gotlib, 2002). Careful study of the functioning of these offspring may therefore provide clues about vulnerability mechanisms. Beyond assessing increased risk factors for the development of a disorder, however, offspring designs can provide a wealth of other data such as whether those offspring who do not emerge with depression will experience risk for some other manner of psychological distress, social difficulties (e.g., impaired peer relationships and social support networks), and academic or vocational difficulties.

Specific Methodological Considerations in Offspring Studies

A number of considerations are essential to offspring designs, some of which are variations on basic research principles, while others are relatively unique to this approach. We summarize these considerations as discussed by Hammen (1991) in her work on the social context of risk in children of depressed mothers.

PARENTAL STATUS

It is important for investigators assessing the children of depressed parents to provide an explicit description of how depression in parents is defined and empirically operationalized. As we have noted, such definitions frequently rely on adherence to DSM criteria, which provide standards not only for inclusion of cases but also for the exclusion of cases (e.g., bipolar disorder, schizophrenia). Explicit operational definitions also allow for the inclusion of comparison groups. For example, to control for hospitalization and family disruption, Hammen (1991) employed the offspring of medically ill patients as a control group in a study of the children of depressed mothers.

The demographic and psychological characteristics of parent samples are also important to assess. As Hammen (1991) notes, many studies combine mothers and fathers without reporting which (or if both) parent(s) met the depression criteria. Whether a father versus a mother is depressed may significantly influence vulnerability of the children to developing depression (see Phares, 1996; Phares & Compas, 1992; Phares, Fields, Kamboukos, & Lopez, 2005). Likewise, if both parents are depressed, the chances of being vulnerable to depression may be considerably enhanced, akin to an additive or perhaps even multiplicative effect.

Comorbidity with depression should also be addressed in offspring studies. For instance, a depressed parent who also evidences a personality disorder may differ in the likelihood of producing at-risk children than a depressed parent without a personality disorder. In this same vein, other psychiatric characteristics are important to examine in offspring studies, such as acute versus chronic disorder, the severity of the disorder, past psychiatric history, and so on. Such characteristics may interact significantly with the development of vulnerability to depression. Likewise, demographic characteristics such as parents' age, socioeconomic status, education level, and ethnicity may also serve as important correlates of the development of vulnerability.

OFFSPRING STATUS

The same precision that is needed to adequately assess parents in offspring studies is also needed to adequately assess children. As with parents, the demographic and psychological characteristics (e.g., age, sex, ethnicity, severity of problems) are also important to consider in offspring. More generally, the interaction between the characteristics of parents and the characteristics of their children in these studies may provide important information about the development of vulnerability.

ASSESSMENT OF MEDIATIONAL VARIABLES FOR BOTH CHILDREN AND PARENTS

Although diagnostic and demographic status in offspring studies can provide important information, this information is limited in its ability to elucidate potential causal relationships; such data are generally only able to provide information about the correlates of vulnerability, but not the actual mechanisms of vulnerability. Demonstrating, for example, that the children of depressed mothers are more likely to develop depression does little to reveal *why* this is the case. This is true even if a particular casual theory predicts that offspring will be at increased risk for the disorder. For example, a theory might predict that offspring are more likely to develop depression because of the transmission of genetic vulnerability factors. However, the mere fact that children are more likely to experience depression does not confirm the operation of the predicted genetic mechanism, nor does it rule out that other factors are involved. Perhaps the proposed genetic mechanism does play a role, but only in combination with another biological process, or perhaps only when dysfunctional communication patterns between disordered parents and child are also present. Offspring studies should thus carefully consider including the assessment of mediating variables that might be hypothesized to provide the crucial links between offspring and vulnerability.

Advantages and Limitations

Offspring studies have the clear advantage of allowing for the assessment of vulnerability processes from a very early point in individuals' history. To the extent that this history is as important as many investigators strongly suggest that it is (Dodge, 1993; Garber, 2010), then assessment of these factors provides a crucial opportunity to begin to understand vulnerability. More specifically, the careful inclusion of mediating variables in study designs provides an opportunity to gain a glimpse of some potential causal mechanisms. Indeed, the call for assessing mediational variables (e.g., Hammen, 1991) addresses exactly this issue and the fact that these designs allow investigators to assess mediational variables in an at-risk sample is a clear advantage of offspring designs.

Some of the limitations of this approach for assessing vulnerability are determined by the age range of the vulnerable people in which investigators are interested. Many designs that are useful for understanding distal vulnerability emanate from research paradigms that are intended to study childhood depression factors. Considerably fewer limitations of these designs are apparent for investigators who seek to understand childhood depression; investigators are able to select vulnerable subjects in an age range that corresponds to their level of interest. That is, because the age of the depression risk that is studied is closer to the ultimate target of interest (depression in children and perhaps adolescents), offspring studies may yield important clues about causal variables at this stage in life.

However, for investigators interested in the distal vulnerability factors that lead to adult depression, this design in and of itself may offer considerably more limited utility. Because offspring studies are typically cross-sectional, they are unable to take into account the almost certain reality that risk processes occurring early in life are affected by a plethora of developmental and social processes that occur as children mature into adults. This is also true even for offspring studies that seek to study the adult offspring of depressed parents. Hence, to place knowledge obtained from offspring studies in a context that is valuable for understanding adult depression, these factors must be assessed over time. While offspring studies therefore constitute a good starting point, to understand distal factors that operate in adult depression they must be combined with longitudinal research strategies.

Another potential limitation is that the sample chosen for offspring studies may be aberrant with regard to the factors that typically operate in the disorder. For example, while the children of depressed parents are in fact at increased risk for depression and other psychological problems (Hammen, 1991), many do not develop depression, and certainly many individuals develop depression whose parents do not have diagnosable psychopathology. By definition, offspring studies are limited to studying samples of depressed parents and their children, and thus important factors may be missed by not assessing nondepressed parents and their children who eventually become depressed. Some of these parents may suffer from other kinds of disorders, but many may not show any evidence of a psychiatric disorder at all.

High-Risk Parental Designs

If the offspring design suggests that it is informative to study the offspring of depressed parents, the reverse is also certainly true—that is, studying the parents of depressed children may also provide important information. The same methodological considerations that apply to offspring designs also apply to parental designs (e.g., careful consideration of not only the descriptive characteristics of depressed children and their parents, but also the inclusion of the assessment of theoretically determined mediational variables for both children and their parents).

The value of the high-risk parental approach can perhaps best be considered within the context of comparisons to offspring designs. For example, the interactions between depressed parents and their at-risk children, and the interactions of nondepressed parents and their at-risk children, may differ in ways that provide clues as to why some children of depressed parents do not become depressed and why some children of nondepressed parents do become depressed. Additionally, the "kind" of depression (e.g., cognitive subtype vs. noncognitive subtype) that is elicited by depressed parents may differ from the "kind" that may be linked to nondepressed parents. This recognizes the heterogeneity of depression (see Chapter 1) and suggests the possibility that depression may have different causal pathways when linked to depressed versus nondepressed parents. Is it possible, for instance, that there is a larger genetic component in the depression suffered by the children of depressed parents than that suffered by the children whose parents are not depressed? Answers to these questions will not be forthcoming until more heterogeneous parental characteristics and behavioral patterns (spanning from psychopathological to relatively healthy) are studied.

Longitudinal Designs

Before examining different types of longitudinal designs, it is important to note that the methodological considerations that we discussed in reference to other designs apply equally to longitudinal designs. That is, explicit operational definitions and assessment of diagnostic, psychological, and demographic status of samples as well as the assessment of mediational variables are critical to consider if longitudinal designs are to yield useful information about distal risk. Moreover, additional considerations frequently need to be taken into account (e.g., developmental stages, ages, sex differences). For a discussion of the issues to evaluate in conducting longitudinal research, see Rutter (2009) and the timeless volume assembled by Rutter (1988).

Theoretical and Empirical Guiding Considerations in Longitudinal Risk Research

In principal, longitudinal research can be atheoretical in that investigators interested in distal vulnerability can administer a large number of measures, follow an unselected group of subjects over time, and then determine which variables predict the occurrence of depressive symptomatology. Large-scale epidemiological studies tend to follow this strategy. In practice, however, for most investigators such a strategy is impractical and far too expensive to yield a sufficient number of participants who will eventually develop depression to learn anything meaningful about the disorder. Instead, longitudinal research is almost always theoretically or empirically driven.

THEORETICAL CONSIDERATIONS

Specific theoretical considerations are frequently employed to help guide the choice of samples to be studied and measures to be used in longitudinal studies. In Chapter 5 we examine the Temple–Wisconsin Cognitive Vulnerability to Depression Project (Alloy, Abramson, Safford, & Gibb, 2006) in more detail. Here we note its relevance as an example of a theory-driven choice of variables. In particular, the theoretical framework of this project specifies the need to obtain measures of participants' attributional tendencies and dysfunctional attitudes.

EMPIRICAL GUIDING CONSIDERATIONS

Empirically observing a relationship between a variable and vulnerability to depression is another way to find clues about which samples and variables to study. For instance, the observation that stress is linked to the onset of depression (see Monroe, 2008; Monroe & Simons, 1991) constitutes sufficient reason in and of itself to study this variable in longitudinal research. In this case, while perhaps desirable, a guiding theoretical framework is unnecessary for the construct of this research (although once adequately documented, theories and data specifying the reasons *why* stress is linked to depression will be needed). Ideally, longitudinal designs will include both empirical and theoretical guiding ideas.

Types of Longitudinal Designs

Several types of longitudinal designs can be employed to study distal vulnerability factors (for an extensive discussion of these longitudinal designs, see Rutter, 1988b). These designs consist of (1) register designs, (2) catch-up designs, (3) follow-back designs, and (4) prospective designs.

REGISTER DESIGNS

As the name suggest, register designs rely on registries of relevant information to assess longitudinal questions. The high-risk studies using Denmark's National Psychiatric Register and the Folkeregister (Kety et al., 1968; Mednick & Schulsinger, 1968; Rosenthal et al., 1968) represent an example of this approach. Thus if an investigator wishes to assess the children of depressed individuals to search for risk factors, he or she could employ a register to help locate these offspring and then ask them questions that may shed light on risk. This is an appealing design if a register is available, but such registers are limited to a very small number of countries and out of reach of the vast majority of investigators.

CATCH-UP DESIGNS

Catch-up designs make use of data previously collected for another purpose to assess a given variable. For example, data relevant to risk that may have been collected when individuals in the sample were young can be examined at a later date to determine if these data predict depressive symptomatology. A study reported by Zuroff et al. (1994) serves as a case in point. This study examined data from a study of 5-year-olds first reported in 1957 by Sears, Maccoby, and Leven. When the sample was age 12, data on self-criticism were collected, and later, when the sample was 18 and 31, data were collected on interpersonal relationships, achievement, and general adjustment. Although data on depression were not collected for this sample, a catch-up design would assess depression (both current and past) and determine whether any of the variables collected earlier, for different purposes, predicted later depression.

FOLLOW-BACK DESIGNS

Follow-back designs reflect the near opposite of catch-up designs. Whereas a catch-up design makes use of previously collected data for individuals in a sample, follow-back designs assess individuals on a particular variable and then search for data that may have been collected earlier that may help understand the variable. A good example can be seen in school records: Can a variable in vulnerable individuals' school records be identified that is correlated with risk?

PROSPECTIVE DESIGNS

Prospective designs identify variables thought to be linked to vulnerability in individuals, and then follow individuals over time to determine if these variables do in fact predict depression. The Temple–Wisconsin Cognitive Vulnerability to Depression Project represents an example of this design, as do two studies reported by Segal et al. (1999, 2006). In these studies, cognitive reactivity in response to a mood induction was assessed in depressed patients who were treated to remission and followed over the course of a number of months. The idea underlying these studies was to determine whether prospectively assessed reactivity would predict relapse. We discuss these results more thoroughly in Chapter 5, but the short answer here is that it did.

Advantages and Limitations

The advantages of longitudinal designs to study risk are considerable. For example, the ability to demonstrate the necessary prerequisite of temporal antecedence (Garber & Hollon, 1991) for determining vulnerability and causality is a fundamental aspect of many longitudinal designs, and is the case particularly for prospective designs. As such, to the extent that temporal antecedence can be demonstrated and shown to be correlated with study variables, such designs can provide powerful inferences about risk. Such designs, again particularly prospective designs, also allow for the relatively precise assessment of critical events, and the assessment of variables that coincide with these events that play a role in the development of vulnerability to depression. Longitudinal designs also allow for the analysis of subgroups (e.g., groups who develop depression and those who do not), as well as the risk variables that potentially differentiate these groups.

From a purely methodological perspective, the limitations of longitudinal studies are relatively few. One methodological problem, however, may result from individuals being tested on more than one occasion (particularly in prospective designs), raising the possibility that repeated testing will alter subsequent test results by creating reactive assessment (see Kazdin, 1992, 2003).

From a practical point of view, the limitations of longitudinal designs are substantial. Given the complexity of issues to be addressed over some period of time, longitudinal designs are difficult to adequately conduct. To justify the effort, time, and expense required to construct a longitudinal vulnerability study, considerable care is needed to ensure adequate representation of variables in the study. The difficulty of this task is likely to be exponentially magnified by the length of the study period. Longitudinal designs are also vulnerable to problems in the collection of data such as high drop-out rates for research participants in prospective designs. Longitudinal research is thus not for the faint-of-heart, researchers without adequate funding, or the untenured.

Cross-Sequential Designs

Cross-sequential designs are derived from developmental psychology research aimed at assessing developmental changes over time (Vasta, Haith, & Miller, 1992), and in structure reflect a combination of longitudinal and cross-sectional research. As in cross-sectional designs, different cohorts are selected for study, and as in longitudinal designs, these different cohorts are followed over some period of time. A number of comparisons are possible from this design. To illustrate a classic cross-sequential design, for instance, groups of 2-year-olds might be studied along with groups of 4-year-olds and 6-year-olds. Several types of comparisons can be made. First are the cross-sectional comparisons; 2-year-olds are compared to 4-year-olds and 2-year-olds and 4-year-olds are compared to 6-year-olds. Second, longitudinal comparisons can also be done so that each cohort is assessed after a specified interval. Thus, for example, the changes that have occurred in the 2-year-old group after 4 years (now 6-year-olds) can be evaluated. Third, and unique to this type of design, cross-sectional/longitudinal comparisons can also be done; after 2 years the original 4-year-old cohort can now be compared with the original 2-year-old cohort (which has now turned 4 years old). In theory there are few limits as to the number of cohorts that can be studied, although practical constraints will reduce this to a number that the investigators deem practically manageable.

Advantages and Limitations

Such designs are applicable in a variety of settings, but are ideal for the study of possible risk variables in children. Moreover, cross-sequential designs compensate for many of the design limitations of cross-sectional studies. In the case of offspring designs, for example, cross-sectional designs are unable to account for how vulnerability processes related to depressed parents are affected by the intervening developmental and social influences that occur over a period of time. Most generally, a well-designed cross-sequential study provides a powerful method for beginning to understand critical aspects of various processes as they pertain to the development of depression. Cross-sequential designs can also be used to assess whether individuals are affected by repeated testing, an issue that cannot be readily resolved in longitudinal designs. As with longitudinal designs, the limitations of cross-sequential designs stem from practical considerations such as the amount of time necessary to track meaningful processes.

Retrospective Designs

Retrospective designs seek to understand the influence of risk factors by examining the recall of information during the time that these factors were thought to be operating. In adults, this entails asking individuals to recall earlier events (from childhood or adolescence) that the investigator hypothesizes might be related to depression. To the extent that information about these possible distal risk factors can be adequately and reliably gathered, they provide a potentially important means for understanding the association of these variables with adult depression. For example, the recall of traumatic events (e.g., abuse; Kuyken & Brewin, 1995; Rose & Abramson, 1995) proposed to be linked to vulnerability may be sought as a way to understand the effects of these events on the development of depression in adults. As another example, if certain parenting behaviors are proposed to be linked to depression vulnerability, then recall of these behaviors would be assessed in retrospective studies (Brewin, Firth-Cozens, Furnham, & McManus, 1992; Gerlsma, Emmelkamp, & Arrindell, 1990; Kuyken & Brewin, 1995).

Retrospective designs may also help understand the link between proximal and distal vulnerability factors. For example, Brewin et al. (1992) reported an association between recalled dysfunctional parenting (a factor potentially related to distal vulnerability) and excessive self-criticism as an adult (a potentially proximal risk factor). Because distal vulnerability probably represents the foundation from which proximal vulnerability is developed, assessing the relationship between distal and proximal vulnerability is important for understanding how people become depressed.

Experimental Retrospective Designs

While the typical retrospective design assesses risk by examining the recall of early experiences by (typically) depressed individuals, experimental retrospective designs can impose experimental conditions to examine somewhat different questions. These experimental conditions in the literature thus far have pertained primarily to priming paradigms, although other experimental procedures are possible. Several priming variations are possible.

Primed recall of distal vulnerability permits assessment of the recall of possible distal vulnerability factors. For instance, disrupted parental bonding experiences have been hypothesized to serve as a vulnerability factor for depression, yet such interactions may not be readily recalled when nondepressed but high-risk individuals are assessed. It is possible, however, that the examination of recollections under priming conditions may facilitate recall. That is, vulnerable individuals who have been primed may be more able to recall these disrupted interactions. It is, of course, also possible that this procedure biases recollections, particularly if the priming condition is one of an induced negative mood. Nevertheless, in principle such a procedure has the potential to generate data that might not otherwise be available.

Advantages and Limitations

A clear advantage of retrospective designs is that they provide access to data on early experiences that may constitute distal vulnerability factors. Moreover, they do so without the expense and logistical difficulties involved in conducting longitudinal research. However, these designs are also vulnerable to criticisms that retrospective reports are likely to be unreliable and thus invalid. Brewin, Andrews, and Gotlib (1993) provided a detailed review of these concerns and classified concerns into three categories: normal limitations in memory, memory deficits associated with psychopathology, and mood-congruent memory processes. However, based on their review of the literature, Brewin et al. (1993) argued that data generally do not substantiate these concerns. For example, while changes in memory do take place over time, data suggest that individuals have fairly good recall of salient facts, which in turn contributes to relatively good recall of the general aspects of events. Nevertheless, Brewin et al. (1993) offer several suggestions to strengthen the validity of these data sources. To the degree possible, they suggest that supplementing retrospective reports with information from other informants can lead to a more valid picture of childhood events, although they caution against parents serving as these other informants because their accounts of events are almost always more positive than their children's. Siblings may provide a better informant group, ideally from same-sexed, similar-aged siblings. Brewin et al. (1993) also suggest that carefully structuring the fashion in which recall is assessed can improve the validity of these reports.

METHODS OF COGNITIVE NEUROSCIENCE

Having examined the kinds of designs used in the study of vulnerability, and in the process of having also illustrated clinically applied methods from cognitive psychology, we turn now to an examination of the methods of cognitive neuroscience. These methods build on the foundations of cognitive psychology and include electrophysiological experiments, neuroimaging, neuropsychology, and behavioral neuroscience. Cognitive neuroscience also makes contact with low-level data from psychophysiological studies of neural systems and, increasingly, cognitive genomics. Before providing a short review of the tools available, it seems pertinent to discuss the general empirical approach often adopted by most scientists in this domain.

The general framework of most cognitive neuroscience research includes both psychological variables and physiological variables that can act as both the independent variable and the dependent variable. The most common case is that the independent variable is something that leads to a concurrent psychological and physiological change.

Examples might include an environmental stimulus that leads to some kind of perception and or response, experimental task demands that lead to one or more cognitive process, or an environmental or internally produced stressor. With regard to the dependent variable, again both psychological variables and physiological variables can act as the dependent variable. However, the most ideal case is if a researcher can measure multiple dependent variables, preferably at least one that is psychological and one that is physiological in nature. A common combination of variables might be reaction times and electrophysiological responses. One concern is that these dependent variables may not always suggest the same conclusions, although this complication can also be theoretically informative.

To provide background information to help clarify subsequent discussions of the application of cognitive neuroscience methods to address specific questions regarding vulnerability to depression, a very brief review of the more commonly used cognitive neuroscience tools is provided here. It is important to point out that methods and related research discussed here focus on "dry physiology." In other words, cognitive neuroscientists tend to rely on methods that can be preformed via noninvasive measurement techniques. Second, for the purposes of the current discussion, we focus on tools that measure central nervous system functions and processes. There are a very large and well-established set of methods that allow for the measurement of more peripheral nervous system functions, classically referred to as "psychophysiological measures," which include measures of skin conductance (skin conductance response, galvanic skin response), cardiovascular measures (heart rate, beats per minute, or heart rate variability), muscle activity (electromyography [EMG]), changes in pupil diameter (pupillometry), and eye movements recorded via the electro-oculogram. We do not directly talk about this category of methods in the current review, although we recognize the utility of these methods for the study of depression.

The cognitive neuroscience methods reviewed here vary in some critical ways. One of the most important skills necessary for a researcher in this area is to know what methods are most appropriate for a given empirical question. Two critical parameters that must be considered is the method's time window of measurement (milliseconds–minutes), also referred to as the method's temporal acuity or temporal resolution, and also the spatial resolution possible with a tool. The time window of measurement is a critical tool for all types of cognitive neuropsychological tools because, when considering how these methods might help us to better understand depression vulnerability, one must consider tonic physiological measures, which might reflect ongoing individual difference variables that might be related to trait-like vulnerability factors. Concurrently, there are also a wide range of phasic or more temporally concise kinds of measures that one might use. These tools also vary in that they require quite different laboratory settings (ambulatory to extreme muscular demobilization) and in a related vein they can be variable with regards to the research population that are best studied with the tool (e.g., it would be inappropriate to use positron emission tomography [PET] with a young child or infant, while it is very common to do electrophysiological research with young children). It is, in part, the consideration of all of these parameters that leads to the range of cognitive neuroscience research that is routinely done.

Within the literature on emotion and depression, the cognitive neuroscience methods that are most commonly used tend to allow insight into broad response systems that Lang and colleagues (e.g., Bradley & Lang, 2000) have called the "emotion output systems." Lang has subdivided the diverse range of emotional responses possible into three broad systems, labeled as *physiological events* (corresponding with the physiological responses that are critical to somatic models of emotion as discussed earlier in this chapter), *language events* (ranging from simple vocal signals like crying to more complex linguistic emotional expressions), and *behavioral events* (either reflecting cognitive or more reflexive goal-directed behaviors). To measure or collect neurophysiological data that provides insight into these three kinds of events, cognitive neuroscientists have employed a range of tools. Below we review three categories of cognitive neuroscience tools that have been effectively applied to the study of emotion, depression, or depression vulnerability. We begin with a class of tools that have the longest history in their application: the electromagnetic tools. After discussing electrophysiological and magnetophysiological measures, a short review covers anatomical imaging and functional imaging tools.

Electrophysiological and Magnetophysiological Methods

This first broad category of cognitive neuroscience tools that will be referred to in the current discussion of the depression vulnerability literature are electrophysiological, electroencephalography (EEG) and event-related potentials (ERPs). There are also a related set of magnetophysiological methods available, though much less research, to date, has been done using these tools. Whenever there is a voltage change due to ionic flow through a neuron cell's membrane, this generates an electrical signal and it generates a magnetic signal. Therefore, EEG and magnetoencephalography (MEG) are effectively sensitive to the same kinds of physiological events, specifically, neuronal activity in the brain. Therefore, because the response system tapped by these tools is the electrocortical activity that is carried out within the neurons themselves, particularly the neurons in the cerebral cortex, they provide a very effective and "direct" tool for measuring depression-related brain functions. Another strength of these tools is their temporal resolution. The frequency of the signals that are most related to cognitive functions are normally less then 30 Hz, and as indicated earlier, the presumed time course of most cognitive processes is such that important physiological changes happen in the time frame of single milliseconds or tens of milliseconds. Even relatively unsophisticated EEG systems can sample electrophysiological activity at a rate of 250–500 Hz, allowing for very effective measurement of behavior-related physiological changes.

One primary limitation of EEG techniques and some applications of ERPs is that the spatial resolution is quite poor. It is mathematically impossible to reconstruct a unique model of the likely current source for an EEG signal. Electrical currents are distorted because the primary current that is generated by the cognitive process that we wish to study can cause secondary currents that are not associated with neuron activity but they look like primary (cellular-generated) currents. When we measure the electrical activity at the scalp, we measure both primary and secondary currents. Electrical currents are also distorted because the brain and skull tissues are not uniform in their conductive properties. The tissue itself distorts the signal. Both of these problems make it very difficult to determine where in the head the electrical signal is coming from (the inverse problem). Thus, when we consider the general goals of functional localization that unite the fields of cognitive psychology and cognitive neuroscience, it might seem that EEG techniques would be of limited use. However, two technological changes mitigate this concern. First, recent development in EEG technology has lead to the growing use of high-density EEG systems. These high-density systems allow for the measurement of signals from as many as 256 electrode sites, which allows for a far more precise estimation of the cortical source of the signal.

Neuronal electrocortical activity not only produces measurable electrophysiological waves at the scalp, but it also produces magnetophysiological waves. Some of the first measurements of biomagnetic activity were centered around measuring magnetic signals being given off by the heart muscle. The inverse problem is much less severe for MEG. In the skull, primary currents do not give rise to significant secondary currents that can distort the signal at the scalp. Magnetic currents are also much less affected by the conductive properties of the tissue they are passing through. Therefore, the result is a less distorted signal at the scalp. Because the signal is less distorted it is easier to try to estimate where the signal is coming from because we can know how the signal is radiating from the cortical source.

When analyzing both EEG and MEG data, one of the most common approaches for interpreting this kind of physiological data is to look for an evoked response or an ERP. Both EEG and MEG necessarily concurrently measure both neuronal activity that is of interest (e.g., the neuronal activity that might be associated with a depressed participant processing a frowning face) and other neuronal signals that are being generated by the myriad of both cognitive and general physiological processes that the brain is executing. Looking for an evoked response is therefore challenging because there is always this "signal-to-noise" problem, the *signal* being the physiological activity tied to the cognitive process of interest and the *noise* being general brain activity. Thus, to see the signal of interest the experimenter must conduct many trials (commonly between 25 and 200) and average the results together, causing random brain activity to be averaged out and the relevant evoked responses or ERPs to become visible. Despite these methodological concerns, cognitive neuroscientists have discovered many different cognitive processes that elicit reliable ERPs from participants. The timing of these responses is thought to provide a measure of the timing of information processing, while the magnitude or amplitude of the evoked responses are thought to reflect something about either the effectiveness of some cognitive process or the resource load that the cognitive process might require.

As with the other methods described above, these methods that provide a measure of cortical electrophysiological activity have been used extensively both to examine stable characteristics of depression and abnormal phasic responses. A more complete discussion is provided in Chapter 6 of work by researchers such as Richard Davidson, Jack Nitschke, Greg Miller, and Wendy Heller who have done a good deal to characterize particular persistent patterns of lateralized EEG activity that might not only be effective at identifying currently depressed individuals (Davidson, 1998, 2000; Heller & Nitschke, 1997; Miller & Cohen, 2001), but also may act as a physiologically marked diathesis (Davidson & Fox, 1989; Dawson, Panagiotides, Klinger, & Spieker, 1997; Field, Diego, & Hernandez-Reif, 2006; Henriques & Davidson, 1990). Just as readily, these electrophysiological tools have been used to examine phasic, cognitively elicited responses as well. One example of this kind of research comes from the study of changes in attentional mechanisms that may be associated with depression. Depression is typically associated with a decrease in the overall amplitude of a component called the P3 or P300, when this ERP signal is being generated by affectively neutral stimuli such as simple nonverbal sounds (e.g., Ancy, Gangadhar, & Janakiramaiah, 1996). On the other hand, there is mounting evidence indicating that depressed individuals display elevated P3s in response to negative information on certain cognitive tasks (Ilardi, Atchley, Enloe, Kwasny, & Garratt, 2007; Ohira, 1996). Thus, this kind of neuropsychological information is thought to provide insight into more persistent cognitive weakness, such as possible selective attention deficits that might play a role in the onset of depression. Additionally, situation-specific cognitive effects associated with depression, such as a hypersensitivity to stimuli that carry negative emotional cues or that might be exceptionally personally self-referential, can be observed. Though we are not aware of any direct evidence to date that has shown that these electrophysiologically manifested depression characteristics, reflected in P3 amplitude, are a direct diathesis for depression, it is clear that this kind of work both could and should be done in the future.

Anatomical Imaging Methods

The primary goal of anatomical imaging is get a very precise image or a "map" of the gross anatomical structures of the body and, more specifically in the literature that we will discuss, in the brain. In a hospital setting, anatomical imaging is generally a part of the discipline of radiology and it involves both the acquisition of anatomical images and the interpretation of these images for purposes of diagnosis and clinical intervention. For example, in a clinical domain imaging might be used to understand where a lesion is located, while in a more research context this tool would allow for comparisons between the anatomy of populations of interest (older vs. younger adults, across gender, across diagnostic groups, etc). In contrast, functional imaging is more like other techniques discussed thus far, which is to understand the physiological changes that correlate with changes in behavior or cognitive processing. At first glance, it might seem that methods that provide reasonable temporal resolution would be necessary to understand the dynamic processes and behaviors that underlie the experience of depression. However, many theories, such as Beck's cognitive theory (see Chapter 5) argue that depression is characterized by trait-like characteristics that influence cognition and behavior. Presumably these persistent functional characteristics would be correlated with relatively tonic or stable physiological characteristics that might be manifested in a patient's gross anatomy. Moreover, given that this text is particularly interested in finding evidence of cognitive and neurocognitive markers that precede the onset of depression, anatomical imaging seems a very fruitful additional tool to consider.

To be able to compare these tools to the others reviewed, consider some of the basic parameters of anatomical imaging. First, anatomical images of the brain normally have no temporal component as a dependent variable. They can be used to monitor changes over time—for example, they can be used to monitory physiological changes in the areas that are being impacted by some kind of damage (e.g., during recovery from a stroke). In general, anatomical imaging provides a static picture of the present anatomy. Furthermore, anatomical imaging can be used in conjunction with other techniques, such as ERP or functional magnetic resonance imaging (fMRI), to provide an image with high spatial resolution over which functional data is superimposed. In this way, anatomical imaging can be used in conjunction with other cognitive neuroscience tools to lend its advantage in spatial clarity to the consideration of functional data that has some degree of temporal resolution.

Many consider autopsy to be the original anatomical imaging method because it provides a static representation of anatomy with high spatial resolution, and because it is used for many of the same purposes as other anatomical imaging tools. Thinking of autopsy this way helps illustrate the strengths and weaknesses of this set of tools. Anatomical imaging that is appropriate for living participants includes tools that rely primarily on x-ray, ultrasound, or electromagnetic technologies. The two most commonly reported kinds of anatomical data come either from computed tomographic (CT) techniques or from magnetic resonance imaging (MRI). CT scans (originally called computerized axial tomographic, or CAT, scans) are computer-analyzed x-ray images. First, the x-ray tube is rotated 360 degrees around the patient, and then the images are processed by a computer in such a way that the computer constructs the image of a "slice" through the brain. The CT scanner will take several scans short distances apart and stack the slices to produce a three-dimensional representation of the brain's anatomy. MRI relies on a very different kind of technology. In order to do magnetic imaging three magnetic fields are needed within the scanner. First a powerful static field is utilized; the "size" of the magnet can range from 0.5 tesla to at least 4.5 tesla for anatomical or functional imaging uses. The second magnetic field is a radio frequency electromagnetic field that produces a pulse sequence. Different pulse sequences make different kinds of tissue more easily seen in the image (e.g., water vs. fat) because different kinds of tissue have different relaxation times. Finally a gradient field is used. This field, generated by a series of coils that circle within the larger permanent, static field, aids in the localization of the signal within the static field. In this way we can build the desired map of the scanned anatomy. While modern CT provides good spatial resolution that is comparable to the spatial precision provided by MRI, MRI provides far better contrast resolution or contrast detail (i.e., the ability to distinguish the differences between two similar but not identical tissues). This difference between CT and MRI likely explains why much of the research we will discuss in Chapter 7 utilizes MRI technologies.

Functional Imaging Methods

Probably the most commonly discussed tools in the arsenal of cognitive neuroscience are the neuroimaging techniques, particularly the functional imaging methods. For the purposes of discussion in the current text this category of research methods would include techniques such as fMRI, PET, single photon emission computed tomography (SPECT), and optical imaging methods. It should be noted that there is an inherent bias in the current review: though we focus more heavily on the application of fMRI, it should be noted that particularly PET imaging has also been a mainstay in the cognitive neuroscience research domain, and research employing this method has made substantial contributions in terms of task development and the development of general functional imaging experimental design. Additionally, for the last 30 years at least, PET methods have been used very effectively as a way to better understand the neurochemical underpinnings of depression and depression vulnerability (for examples, see Mayberg et al., 1988; Meyer et al., 1999, 2003; Yatham, Liddle, & Shiah, 2000). The decision to focus more heavily on fMRI studies in part stems from the goal of the current review, which is to primarily discuss research that sheds light on the emotion output systems as outlined by Lang above (specifically physiological events, language events, and behavioral events).

When researches first started applying these tools it was suggested that these methods might easily make all other neuropsychology related methods fundamentally obsolete because these tools could provide a map with high spatial resolution indicating all the brain regions recruited for a given cognitive task. This turned out to be an overly rosy prognosis regarding the utility of these tools. Nonetheless, their contribution to the field has been significant. Functional imaging methods primarily allow us to see physiological responses during behavior. They are not designed to provide good anatomical pictures, but instead they allow us to observe different kinds of physiological markers such as regional changes in glucose metabolism, regional changes in blood oxygenation, or changes in reflected infrared light that are related to blood oxygenation. These tools are, again, best known for their relatively high spatial resolution; recent technological advances have improved spatial resolution to the millimeter scale. The degree of temporal resolution varies significantly between methods, with PET being the worst (minute-level resolution) and some optical imaging having some of the best temporal resolutions, comparable to electroencephalography and magnetoencephalography (with millisecond-level resolution). These imaging tools allow us to either compare the physiological state of the brain at time 1 versus time 2 or they can be used to watch the whole time course of a physiological/ behavioral response.

Regarding the response system being measured, functional imaging tools most often measure hemodynamic or metabolic activity with the cardiovasculature of the brain. Thus, the central nervous system is the primary focus of these tools, though the peripheral nervous system certainly does introduce noise into the hemodynamic signal being measured. A concern with functional imaging that results from the response system being measured is related to the fact that cardiovascular change is a slow or lagging indicator of functional change. It takes about 2 seconds for an area to start getting more blood once the neuronal tissue in the area becomes more active, and this change in blood flow lasts for at least 8 seconds. But it takes less then a second to do most cognitive tasks (e.g., about 300–350 msec to read a word). Thus, even with technological improvements in imaging, the response system being measured gives us a delayed and "sluggish" measure of cognition. These characteristics of the response system being measured ultimately reduce the temporal resolution of these tools. However, because of the strong spatial resolution provided by these tools, much can be learned about vulnerability to depression via the application of functional imaging methods.

The application of functional neuroimaging methods to the study of depression vulnerability will often fall into the category of research designed to find more long-term or tonic physiological expressions of the disorder, or designed to help find more phasic responses in depressed or at-risk individuals that are different from the phasic cortical cardiovascular responses seen in never-depressed individuals. A recent example of a depression-related phasic response is a set of fMRI findings that suggest that depressed individuals show greater amygdala activity and hypoactivity of dorsal lateral prefrontal cortex in response to emotion relevant stimuli, such as fear-provoking pictures (Fales et al., 2008; Siegle, Thompson, Carter, Steinhauser, & Thase, 2007). This corticolimbic dopamine system is thought to be involved in general reward processing. Furthermore, it has been argued that abnormalities in this system could underlie the anhedonia which constitutes a major symptom of depression (see Martin-Soelch, 2009, for a review). Functional imaging methods have been aptly applied to examine this dysfunctional dopamine hypothesis (Kumer et al., 2008; Tremblay et al., 2005). Throughout the rest of this book, the methods and assumptions we have discussed will be invoked as we examine cognitive neuroscience research designed to assess vulnerability to depression.

SUMMARY

In this chapter we have provided a description of the basic methods used in the study of vulnerability. Thus, we examined the distinction between proximal and distal vulnerability, and assessed the research designs used to examine these different points on the vulnerability perspective. For example, we noted that proximal designs have employed cross-sectional studies, remission designs, and priming designs. For distally oriented research, we examined high-risk offspring designs, the less well-studied high-risk-parental designs, longitudinal designs, and cross-sectional designs. We also examined the advantages and disadvantages of each, and discussed the issues involved in their use in the study of depression vulnerability.

The methods of cognitive vulnerability are reasonably well known, and their description was thus imbedded in the discussion of various research designs. Owing to their relative "newness" in psychology, and to their greater complexity, we examined cognitive neuroscience methods separately. Our review was divided into three categories. The first category discussed includes EEG and MEG methods. These tools are sensitive to neuronal activity in the brain. Therefore, because the response system tapped by these methods is the electrocortical activity that is carried out within the neurons themselves, particularly the neurons in the cerebral cortex, they provide a very effective and "direct" tool for measuring potential vulnerability-related brain functions. The second category was anatomical imaging methods, whose primary goal is to obtain a very precise image or a "map" of the gross anatomical structures of the brain. Finally, functional neuroimaging methods were examined as a way to look for the long-term physiological expressions of depression vulnerability, or they can be used to study how the responses made by depressed or at-risk individuals differ from the physiological responses seen in never depressed individuals. These three categories of methods allow for the observation of the functions of our nervous system and other physiological response systems that can add to our understanding of both normal behavior, depression, and depression vulnerability.

5

Theory and Data
on Cognitive Vulnerability

Neuroscience research is rich in theory, but owing to a fairly long theoretical history in depression, cognitive vulnerability research tends to be driven somewhat more by theory than is research in neuroscience. That is, the vast majority of cognitive research springs from firmly established cognitive depression theories, and has aimed in a general sense to test the ideas embedded in these theories. Thus, in this chapter, we summarize these theoretical models, and do so for both proximal vulnerability perspectives and distal vulnerability perspectives. We start in a very broad sense by briefly reviewing the diathesis–stress idea, and then examine proximal vulnerability theory and research. We next move to a more distal focus and discuss theory and data on distal cognitive vulnerability.

DIATHESIS–STRESS INTERACTIONS
IN COGNITIVE MODELS OF DEPRESSION

As noted in the diathesis–stress perspective examined in Chapters 2 and 3, under ordinary conditions, the cognitions of who are at risk for depression are indistinguishable from those of the general population. Cognitive models, however, posit that depression is produced by the interaction between a cognitive diathesis and environmental conditions that serve to trigger this diathesis into operation. Hence, when confronted with certain stressors, differences between vulnerable and nonvulnerable people emerge (Monroe & Simons, 1991; Monroe, Slavich, & Georgiades, 2009). As we have noted, for vulnerable people these life events precipitate a pattern of negative, biased, self-referent information processing that appears to initiate the first cycle in the downward spin of depression (Ingram, Miranda, & Segal, 1998; Segal & Shaw, 1986). Nonvulnerable individuals, on the other hand, react with an "appropriate" level of distress and depressive affect to the event, but do not spiral into depression.

An account of these differential outcomes in face of similar life conditions can be found in cognitive models focusing on the dysfunctional cognitive structures and the types of thoughts that come to mind in these situations. For example, Beck (1963, 1967) suggested that schemas about the self are causally linked to the disorder and are triggered by stressful life events. Likewise, Abramson et al. (1989) propose that hopelessness is a sufficient cause of depression in that hopelessness develops in the presence of a negative life event in an important area of the individual's life. When coupled with attributions about the event that are stable, global, and have implications for the person's view of him- or herself, hopelessness depression occurs. Although life events are not specifically highlighted in this model, they are nevertheless critical in that the diatheses in this model is a general tendency to explain events in terms of stable and global causes, to view negative events as having extremely negative consequences, and to see negative events as lowering for self-esteem.

There are hundreds of studies examining schema-driven or attributional-based cognitive processing during the depressed state. As discussed in Chapter 3, however, these data are not typically informative about cognition and depression risk because they do not adequately model the causal complexity of cognitive theories of vulnerability (Hollon, 1992). That is, knowing that a person's thoughts may follow one pattern over another is important, but this line of study does not tell us what serves to activate or set off these thoughts, or under which conditions people will react to cues by employing depressive thinking. This is true for the investigation of distal risk, but this is especially important for accounts of proximal risk factors, since these factors operate in close proximity to the development of depression, and it is important to understand the circumstances that trigger these changes that lead to the depressed state. Thus, cognitive diathesis–stress models remind us that individuals at risk for depression should have latent but reactive negative cognitive structures available that will emerge under certain circumstances. They also remind us that the assessment of cognitive vulnerability should consider strategies capable of activating or priming the reemergence of cognitive variables.

PROXIMAL COGNITIVE RISK RESEARCH

Much, although not all, of the research that pertains to proximal cognitive risk derives from priming research. The use of priming procedures is derived from models that acknowledge that activation occurs in response to a stimulus. Theoretically it makes sense in the lab to model these types of activating features. As a practical matter, however, it is not possible (ethically at least) to create stressful events that mimic the core concerns suggested by Beck's model and the hopelessness model. Rather, studies tend to attempt to create the kind of affective response that accompanies a stressful event, albeit at a very mild level and for a very short duration. Priming studies have thus typically, although not universally, relied on inducing a negative mood in individuals who are presumed to have the requisite vulnerability factors. The extent to which individuals experience negative thinking when evoked with a prime can be thought of as *cognitive reactivity*, the idea that vulnerable individuals react with negative thinking in response to a challenging event.

The cognitive vulnerability research in general, and the priming research in particular, has grown to the point that it does not make efficient use of space to try to describe this research either exhaustively or in great detail. Thus, here we limit ourselves to providing examples of cognitive vulnerability research. We also note at the outset that some studies have been reported that do not support a cognitive vulnerability perspective (e.g., Dykman, 1997) in that they tend to fail to find significant differences between a high-risk group (frequently defined by a previous episode of depression) and a low-risk group (defined by the absence of a previous episode). It is always difficult to interpret null results, but given the wealth of data that have now accumulated (see Scher et al., 2005; Segal & Ingram, 1994), these anomalies do not provide a substantial challenge to conclusions about cognitive vulnerability.

Vulnerability research shares a common set of operational definitions of vulnerability and cognitive processes. As we have discussed, a common operational definition of vulnerability is to study individuals with past experience, or experiences, with depression. Although not perfect, epidemiological data on relapse and recurrence suggest that a significant proportion of these individuals will become depressed again in the future (Boland & Keller, 2009) and that presumably at least a substantial subset of these individuals possess vulnerability factors. Additionally, this research tends to share a common perspective on the kinds of cognitive variables that should be observed in the vulnerability process, although how these variables are operationalized tends to differ to some degree from study to study. For the purposes of our exploration of cognitive vulnerability, we divide these dependent variables into self-report cognitive outcomes and information-possessing-based outcomes.

Cognitive Reactivity

Self-Report Measures of Irrational Beliefs and Dysfunctional Attitudes

Because dysfunctional attitudes constitute a central feature in Beck's (1967, 1987) model of depression, it not a surprise that the Dysfunctional Attitude Scale (Weissman & Beck, 1978) is a common measure in priming studies. Miranda and Persons (1988) reported one of the first studies to assess dysfunctional attitudes and mood, and found that in people who had a history of depression level of mood predicted the endorsement of dysfunctional attitudes. More specifically, they found a linear relationship showing that as negative mood increased, so did the endorsement of more dysfunctional attitudes. Analogous results have been found by the same research group (e.g., Miranda, Gross, Persons, & Hahn, 1988; Miranda, Persons, & Byers, 1990).

Parallel data have been reported by Roberts, Gotlib, and Kassel (1996), Solomon, Haaga, Brody, Kirk, and Friedman (1998), and Gemar et al. (2001). When they examined automatic thoughts, self-esteem, and dysfunctional attitudes, Roberts and Kassel (1996) found stronger relationships between negative affect and these constructs for previously depressed persons than for never depressed persons. In a similar fashion, Solomon et al. (1998) found a stronger association between negative mood and irrational beliefs among recovered depressed persons than among never depressed persons. Gemar et al. (2001) also found that formerly depressed individuals evidenced a greater change in dysfunctional beliefs following a negative mood induction than did never depressed persons.

Segal and colleagues have also examined dysfunctional attitudes in two studies, but included several additional elements. In the first, Segal et al. (1999) assessed a group of formerly depressed patients who had been treated to remission with either cognitive-behavioral therapy or with antidepressants, who following treatment, participated in a mood induction task in which changes in dysfunctional attitudes were examined. Segal et al. (1999) found that when participants were in a normal mood, there was little evidence of dysfunctional attitudes, which was equally true for participants treated with cognitive therapy and participants treated with pharmacotherapy. In the second study, Segal et al. (2006) found similar results. In both studies, however, inducing a sad mood was associated with increased dysfunctional attitudes for the pharmacotherapy group but not for the cognitive therapy group. Hence, patients treated with pharmacotherapy showed significantly greater cognitive reactivity relative to participants treated with cognitive therapy. Moreover, in both studies cognitive reactivity was predictive of depression relapse several years later; patients who responded with fewer dysfunctional attitudes were significantly less likely to relapse compared with patients who reported more dysfunctional attitudes following the sad mood induction. These studies thus show not only a link between vulnerability and the emergence of dysfunctional attitudes, but further suggest that these attitudes are differentially modified by different treatments, and that they are predictive of future depressive episodes.

Information Processing

RECALL

Using a mood induction, Teasdale and Dent (1987) found that recovered depressed persons were more likely to recall negative adjectives endorsed as self-descriptive than were never depressed persons. Likewise, Gilboa and Gotlib (1997) found support for biased recall among formerly dysphoric persons following a negative mood induction. Williams, Watts, MacLeod, and Matthews (1988) also examined recall, specifically, the recall of positive and negative self-referent adjectives under a neutral mood and an induced sad mood. Williams followed participants for a period of a year to determine who experienced a significant episode of depression and found that research participants who recalled more negative than positive self-descriptors in mildly sad mood were more likely to become depressed over that period of time.

Although most priming research relies on mood primes, Hedlund and Rude (1995) examined incidental recall and intrusions of negative and positive words following a self-focus manipulation. This type of prime follows from theory and data on self-focused attention that suggests this process may initiate access to a network of dysfunctional cognitive and affective processes that eventuate in disorder (Ingram, 1990), and, in this case, may characterize risk for depression. Hedlund and Rude found that, when self-focused, formerly depressed persons recalled more negative words and had fewer positive intrusions compared to never depressed persons.

INTERPRETIVE BIASES

In addition to recall, Hedlund and Rude (1995) used a scrambled sentences task to study interpretive biases in depression risk. Results indicated that formerly depressed persons constructed more negative sentences than never depressed persons following the self-focus manipulation. Gemar et al. (2001) also examined self-evaluative bias with a negative mood induction and found that at-risk people evidenced a negative self-evaluative bias following the induction, whereas never depressed individuals did not evidence such a shift. Interestingly, the postinduction negative bias demonstrated by the nondepressed risk group was comparable to that evidenced by a currently depressed group.

ATTENTION

Several studies have examined attentional processes in never depressed and high-risk individuals. For example, using a modified dichotic listening paradigm to assess attention to positive and negative stimuli, Ingram et al. (1994) found that vulnerable individuals devoted attention to both positive and negative stimuli when in a negative mood state. These results were replicated by Ingram and Ritter (2000) who found that vulnerable, but not nonvulnerable individuals, directed attention toward negative stimuli, but only when they were in a negative mood. Unlike the earlier study, however, no effects were found for positive words. Similar results have been reported by McCabe, Gotlib, and Martin (2000).

The Behavioral High-Risk Paradigm

As we noted in Chapter 4, behavioral high-risk paradigms use a theoretically defined, or empirically observed, risk factor to study people who are assumed to possess this risk factor. Although several studies have used this paradigm, we will highlight the arguably predominant high-risk study that provides data on proximal cognitive vulnerability: the Temple–Wisconsin Vulnerability to Depression Project and the depressogenic personality/life stress congruency approach.

The Temple–Wisconsin Project

The Temple–Wisconsin Vulnerability to Depression Project was a two-site, prospective longitudinal study to evaluate the etiological postulates of both the hopelessness model and Beck's theory of depression (Alloy et al., 1996). The idea underlying this project was to assess a group of individuals identified as possessing negative inferential styles, or negative self-schemas, and to compare their outcomes with individuals not showing these cognitive characteristics. Currently nondepressed college freshman were assessed at both Temple University and the University of Wisconsin, and were followed over a 2½-year period. Paralleling the hopelessness theory of depression and Beck's cognitive model, participants were assessed for negative inferential style, that is, the tendency to make self-deprecating attributions for the cause of events, and dysfunctional attitudes, a central feature of Beck's model.

Because the Temple–Wisconsin Vulnerability to Depression Project represents an unusually comprehensive study of vulnerability, we will focus on only the project's major findings with regard to the prediction of depression onset in this sample (for a description of other findings from the project, see Alloy, Abramson, Grant, & Liu, 2009). In particular, the project examined both the onset of major and minor depression, as well as the onset of anxiety disorders, and the theoretically defined idea of hopelessness depression. We examine here only diagnoses of major depression (at least five out of nine depressive symptoms) and minor depression (between two and five symptoms). The high-risk group was found to have significantly more onsets of both major and minor depressive symptoms over the follow-up period (Alloy et al., 2009). Indeed, among high-risk participants, approximately 75% experienced one of these diagnoses over the follow-up period, with major depression accounting for about 23% of cases and minor depression accounting for approximately 52%. Alloy et al. further divided their high-risk group into those who had previously experienced a depressive episode (about 57% of the sample) in order to assess first-onsets verses relapses or recurrences. Not surprisingly, the high-risk group that had previously experienced a depressive episode had a high number of major and minor depression onsets. Indeed, the vast majority of these individuals, approximately 85%, experienced depression. Approximately 62% of the high-risk group with a previous episode experienced major or minor depression. Clearly, possessing the cognitive vulnerability factors outlined by cognitive theories does predict the onset of depression.

Summary of Proximal Risk Research

The data on proximal risk show that priming effects vulnerable individuals in ways that cut across several different levels of cognitive analysis (Ingram, 1990). For instance, in the presence of negative mood, dysfunctional cognition for those at risk appears evident in interpretive biases, cognitive content (i.e., Dysfunctional Attitude Scale [DAS] scores), attention and information encoding, retrieval and memory (adjective recall; Dent & Teasdale, 1988; Hedlund & Rude, 1995; Teasdale & Dent, 1987). Additionally, these processes can predict subsequent episodes of depression. Data from a behavioral high-risk perspective also show evidence that negative cognitions can predict future episodes of depression.

DISTAL COGNITIVE RISK RESEARCH

Theory and research on cognitive vulnerability factors in childhood and adolescent depression are important in their own right, but such perspectives may also provide significant clues about cognitive vulnerability to depression in adults. That is, if distal vulnerability can be conceptualized as the creation of risk in childhood and adolescence, then understanding these processes can be informative about the cognitive factors linked to depression in adults. It is important to note, however, that although important distal risk information may be derived from cognitive conceptual and empirical work with children and adolescents, these are not the only sources of information concerning distal vulnerability. In particular, several theoretical perspectives are informative about distal cognitive risk factors.

Childhood Events in the Creation of Distal Cognitive Vulnerability

Can events in childhood create cognitive risk in adults? Just as there is a substantial body of work showing that adult depression is linked to the occurrence of stressful life events (Monroe & Simons, 1991; Monroe et al., 2009), a considerable body of work also suggests that depression in adulthood is associated with the occurrence of negative events in childhood (Alloy et al., 2001; Garber, 2010). For the purposes of understanding cognitive vulnerability, it is important, however, to examine the *cognitive effects* of such events that may serve to mediate childhood adversity and adult depression. Some conceptual explanations have been offered to establish a bridge between the multitude of negative events in childhood and subsequent adult vulnerability to depression (Goodman & Brand, 2009). We thus turn to a discussion of theoretical models that might guide theorizing about the nature of distal cognitive vulnerability and which may provide a guideline for understanding data that are pertinent to distal vulnerability.

Adult-Based Theories Relevant to Distal Cognitive Vulnerability

The Cognitive Schema Model

Most theoretical discussion devoted to the model originally proposed by Beck in 1967 has been directed toward the development and course of depression in adults (see Engel & DeRubeis, 1993; Haaga et al., 1991; Sacco & Beck, 1995). In a similar fashion, most research that has attempted to test various aspects of the model has been conducted with adults (Haaga et al., 1991). Yet a core feature of this model is the idea that vulnerability to depression develops through the acquisition of cognitive schemas developed during stressful or traumatic events in childhood and adolescence. In particular, Beck argues that when such events occur relatively early in the individual's development, these individuals become sensitized to just these types of events, and when similar events occur in the future (in adulthood for our purposes) these schemas, and corresponding depression, are activated.

> In childhood and adolescence, the depression-prone individual becomes sensitized to certain types of life situations. The traumatic situations initially responsible for embedding or reinforcing the negative attitudes that comprise the depressive constellation are the prototypes of the specific stresses that may later activate these constellations. When a person is subjected to situations reminiscent of the original traumatic experiences, he may then become depressed. The process may be likened to conditioning in which a particular response is linked to a specific stimulus; once the chain has been formed, stim-

uli similar to original stimulus may evoke the conditioned response. (Beck, 1967, p. 278)

Thus, while most commonly viewed as theory of adult depression, Beck's (1967) model specifically and centrally incorporates the conceptual development of distal vulnerability factors.

Hopelessness Depression

Rose and Abramson (1992) were among the first to elaborate upon the developmental antecedents that may underlie the hopelessness theory of depression by suggesting that children who experience negative events seek to find the causes, consequences, and meaning of these events. Rose and Abramson (1992) also suggest that young children have a tendency to make internal attributions for all events, including negative events. Such internal attributional inclinations, however, are by themselves insufficient to lead to a hopelessness attributional style. It is to the extent that unpleasant events are repetitive and occur in the context of relationships with significant others that these events begin to undermine the child's need to maintain both a positive self-image and an optimism about future nonnegative or hopeful events. Moreover, the continuation of such events along with the degradation of positive self-image are hypothesized to produce a pattern of attributions for negative events that tend to be, and become over time, stable and global. Once this inferential pattern for situational contexts becomes more trait-like, the foundation is set for hopelessness responses in the face of future stressors, that are in turn linked to the onset of hopelessness depression.

Distal Cognitive Vulnerability in Developmentally Based Theories

The schema and hopelessness models are focused specifically on adult depression, and as such their accounts of proximal vulnerability are more thoroughly articulated than accounts of distal vulnerability. Several developmentally based models, however, have been developed that highlight what we refer to as distal cognitive vulnerability.

Attachment Theory

Attachment theory addresses variables and processes that shape the capacity of individuals to form meaningful and enduring emotional bonds with significant others throughout their lives (Bowlby, 1969, 1973, 1980). The development of this capacity begins at birth and continues as the child matures. Several investigators have argued that attachment patterns are relatively stable and persist into adulthood (Ainsworth, 1989; Bartholomew & Horowitz, 1991; Doane & Diamond, 1994; Ricks, 1985), and indeed, Bowlby suggested that attachment is a process that extends from "cradle to grave."

The primary determinants of the individual's attachment patterns are thought to be both the quantity and the quality of contact with caretakers (Ainsworth, Blehar, Waters, & Wall, 1978). In particular, consistently nurturant, affectionate, and appropriately protective interactions with caretakers promote the development of the child's ability to form cognitive, behavioral, and emotional connectedness to others. Yet, when normal developmental processes are disrupted, a variety of deviations from secure attachment have been proposed. Theorists suggest that disruptions in the attachment process can result in a variety of insecure attachments labeled "insecure–ambivalent" attachment, "insecure–avoidance" attachment, or "insecure–disorganized" attachment.

These insecure or dysfunctional attachment patterns have been posited to serve as risk factors for a diversity of problems in childhood and beyond (e.g., Bemporad & Romano, 1992; Cummings & Cicchetti, 1990). Of interest for our purposes are the links that have been suggested not only between disrupted attachment and depression, but between these variables and cognitive factors. That is, the risk that originates from dysfunctional attachment patterns may stem from cognitive variables; specifically, theoretical discussions of attachment have emphasized the importance of internal *working models*. These models reflect the cognitive representation of relationships that have been generalized through early interactions with key figures. Attachment theorists propose that once developed, these internal working models guide the processing of information, and the cognitions individuals experience about relationships with others. If attachment is insecure, this will be reflected in the organization and functioning of the individual's working models in ways that lead to an increased risk for stress and disrupted interpersonal functioning as information about interpersonal interactions is distorted (see Bowlby, 1988).

Parental Bonding

Although similar in a number of respects to attachment theory, parental bonding approaches focus on the effects of dysfunctional parenting on depression. This idea may be best illustrated with reference to the instrument that is used to examine bonding, the Parental Bonding Instrument (PBI; Parker, Tupling, & Brown, 1979), which assesses the recall of maternal and paternal caring and overprotectiveness. Care is defined by nurturance and warmth, with low levels of parental care correspondingly being defined as either neglect or by overt rejection. Overprotectiveness, on the other hand, refers to control and intrusiveness. Low levels of care may lead to vulnerability by disrupting the child's self-esteem (Parker, 1979, 1983). Overprotectiveness is thought to operate on vulnerability because the parent is so intrusive that a genuine caring relationship cannot be established with the child. Children who have experienced high levels of overprotectiveness thus do not develop the skills necessary to negotiate successful relationships.

Other dimensions of family interactions may be important for vulnerability, but there is substantial agreement that lack of care and overprotectiveness appear to be core dimensions in the genesis of risk. Blatt and Homann (1992), Burbach and Borduin (1986), and Gerlsma et al. (1990) note the presence of a substantial body of literature showing that disruptions in early interactions with parents are indeed linked to a greater likelihood of experiencing depression. From a cognitive vulnerability standpoint, disruptions in the appropriate level of protectiveness and care by parents are candidates for producing the negative self-structures that are seen in depression risk. Parental bonding may thus be associated with dysfunctional cognitive patterns.

Distal Cognitive Vulnerability Research

Parenting and Early Experiences

A substantial amount of research on distal vulnerability comes from retrospective studies. These studies tend to focus on parental interactions or early abuse experiences and are guided by a variety of theoretical perspectives.

PARENTAL INTERACTIONS

Whisman and Kwon (1992) found that lower levels of parental care were associated with a higher level of depressive symptoms in a mildly depressed sample. More relevant from a cognitive risk perspective, they also found that this relationship was mediated by depressotypic attitudes and dysfunctional attributions. Similar findings have been reported by Roberts, Gotlib, and Kassel (1996) and Whisman and McGarvey (1995), who examined the relationship between cognition, adult attachment, and depressive symptoms and found that attachment levels were associated with depressive symptoms through their effects on dysfunctional attitudes and self-esteem.

From a parental bonding perspective, Ingram, Overbey, and Fortier (2001) found that individuals who report more positive maternal bonding experiences also report more positive and fewer negative thoughts than do those with poor maternal bonding. These results suggest that ambient levels of automatic thinking may explain some of the increased risk experienced by individuals with poor bonding, and also suggest that of the more broadly defined variables, deficits in *maternal* care may be the more specific variable that is linked to dysfunctional cognition. Similar results were reported by Ingram and Ritter (2000) with regard to the specificity of maternal care, an idea that we return to later in this chapter.

Interestingly, there is also some evidence that poorly bonded individuals limit their attention to depressive information as assessed by a Stroop task (Ingram, Bailey, & Siegle, 2004). It is thus possible that although poorly bonded individuals might experience higher "ambient" levels of dysfunctional cognition, their actual information processing occurs in ways that is designed to avoid depressive information. It may be that poorly bonded individuals, who tend to think negatively about themselves, may preattentively seek to regulate their risk by managing information in ways that lead to the minimization of negative information. Explaining a similarly observed avoidance, Gotlib et al. (1988) suggested a "zoom lens" model of attention (Eriksen & Yeh, 1985) to interpret their results to mean that nondepressed individuals may deploy attention that is more constricted, which allows the semantic qualities of information to receive less attention (see also Amir et al., 1996, and Moretti, Segal, McCann, & Shaw, 1996).

Ingram and Ritter (2000) operationalized vulnerability in much the same way that other investigators have done so, specifically by virtue of studying nondepressed individuals who had previously experienced a depressive episode. Results from a dichotic listening task suggested that vulnerable individuals directed attention to negative stimuli when they had been primed by a sad mood. They also found that ratings of maternal care were associated with this attention; specifically, lower reported levels of maternal care were associated with the processing of more negative information when vulnerable individuals were in a negative mood. These data may suggest that a perceived lack of caring by the mother may set the stage for the development of a depressive self-schema. That is, if a parent is unduly critical, or otherwise less than nurturant, the child may assimilate cognitive representations of current or future significant others as hurtful, neglectful, or unreliable, along with developing a cognitive structure that represents the self as unworthy of care (Batagos & Leadbeater, 1995). The development of such structures may be facilitated by sad mood states associated with caretaker interactions, and may be reactivated by subsequent sad mood states whether associated with a caretaker or not.

Several studies have assessed self-criticism as a distally developed cognitive vulnerability factor. For example, McCranie and Bass (1984) found that among nursing students, an overcontrolling mother was associated with greater dependency needs, while for students who had both a mother and a father who were overcontrolling, a greater tendency toward self-criticism was found. Likewise, Brewin et al. (1992) found among young medical students that higher levels of self-criticism were related to reports of inadequate parenting. This was particularly true for individuals who consistently reported high levels of self-criticism over time. Similar results have been reported by Blatt, Wein, Chevron, and Quinlan (1979). Since both dependency and self-criticism have been discussed as possible cognitive (proximal) vulnerability factors, and have been shown in other studies to be associated with depressive states (Blatt & Zuroff, 1992), these data may be relevant for eventually understanding the cognitive diathesis of depression.

EARLY ABUSE EXPERIENCES

Research has suggested a consistent relationship between reports of abusive experiences and depression (Browne & Finkelhor, 1986; Cutler & Nolen-Hoeksema, 1991; Kendall-Tackett, Williams, & Finkelhor, 1993), although only a few studies have examined the cognitive correlates of these experiences (Gibb, 2002). Of those studies investigating negative cognition, the research does support a link between abuse and negative cognitive patterns. For example, Hankin (2005) found that early abuse experiences were associated with depressive symptoms, and that insecure attachment and depressotypic attributions mediated this association. In an earlier study investigating cognitive variables within the context of abuse and depression, Kuyken and Brewin (1995) assessed memory retrieval in a sample of depressed patients, some of whom had experienced sexual and/or physical abuse as children. Kuyken and Brewin's (1995) data indicated that depressed women who had been sexually (but not physically) abused showed an inability to recall specific memories in response to both positive and negative cues, suggesting the possibility that avoidance of key memories and disruptions in working memory may play a role in the relationship between abuse and depression. They also found that parental indifference was related to this inability to recall specific events.

From a different perspective, Rose, Abramson, Hodulik, Halberstadt, and Leff (1994) examined the mediational effect of cognitive variables on the relationship between sexual abuse and depression. In assessing the possibility of different subgroups of depressed individuals, they found that one group who had experienced childhood sexual abuse was characterized by dysfunctional attitudes and attributions. Rose and Abramson (1992) also found that depressed individuals who were maltreated as children had dysfunctional cognitions. Taken together these data suggest that a history of early adverse experiences may produce the distal cognitive patterns that lead toward the later development of depression.

High-Risk Studies

Recall that high-risk offspring studies assess individuals with known or suspected vulnerability. Most, although not all, of the distal risk research examines children with depressed parents. The underlying assumption of this strategy is that offspring are at increased risk for developing a disorder similar to that of one or both of their parents. Although there are a number of possible avenues of vulnerability transmission that have been proposed by vulnerability researchers (e.g., genetic, birth or prebirth trauma) certain interactional patterns involving parents are presumed most likely to lead to the development of vulnerable cognitive structures for depression.

PARENTAL DEPRESSION

Perhaps the most studied vulnerability factor for adult depression has been parental psychopathology. Numerous reviews of the empirical literature leave little doubt that children of depressed mothers are more vulnerable to a variety of difficulties such as interpersonal and academic problems than are children whose mothers are not depressed. Additionally, children of depressed mothers show both an increased incidence of psychological symptoms and increased rates of psychiatric diagnoses, including depression (Beardslee, Bemporad, Keller, & Klerman, 1983; Blatt & Homann, 1992; Cohn & Campbell, 1992; Downey & Coyne, 1990; Gelfand & Teti, 1990; Hammen, 1991; Morrison, 1983; Weissman, 1988). Although data on fathers is noticeably missing in most of these studies (who may play an important role [Phares, 1996; Phares & Compas, 1992]), this line of research nevertheless makes it clear that parental depression is a clear risk factor for offspring depression.

Some research has assessed possible cognitive vulnerability factors in the offspring of depressed parents. For example, in a study examining attributional patterns in conjunction with parental depression, Radke-Yarrow, Belmont, Nottelmann, and Bottomly (1990) found that children of depressed mothers reported higher negative-toned self-attributions than did children of nondepressed mothers. Moreover, mother and child statements were congruent; mothers who endorsed the statement "I hate myself" were likely to have a child who endorsed the statement "I am bad." Garber and Robinson (1997) similarly found evidence of depressotypic attributions and negative automatic thoughts in the children of depressed mothers.

PARENTAL DEPRESSION AND COGNITIVE REACTIVITY

Following from studies assessing cognitive reactivity in high-risk adults, some studies have also assessed cognitive reactivity in the children of depressed mothers. Interpretive bias was examined following a negative mood induction in a study by Dearing and Gotlib (2009), who found that the daughters of depressed mothers interpreted ambiguous words more negatively and less positively than did the daughters of nondepressed mothers. Using a negative mood prime Joormann, Talbot, and Gotlib (2007) examined attention in the children of depressed mothers. Specifically, using an emotional-faces dot-probe task, they found that children of depressed mothers selectively attended to negative facial expressions whereas children of nondepressed mothers attended to positive facial expressions.

In another study assessing cognitive reactivity in the children of depressed mothers, Taylor and Ingram (1999) examined information-processing indices of negative self-schemas in children between the ages of 8 and 12, who had either depressed or nondepressed mothers. Half of the children participated in a mood induction task and the other half participated in a neutral mood induction and then completed the self-referent encoding task. When recall patterns were examined, results showed that negative mood enhanced the recall of negative personally relevant stimuli in high-risk children. Even children as young as 5 years old have been found to evidence these kinds of cognitive patterns. In particular, Murray, Woolgar, Cooper, and Hipwell (2001) assessed children of depressed mothers using an age-appropriate mood induction, and found that these children expressed more hopelessness cognitions than the children of nondepressed mothers. Overall, these data thus suggest that depressed mothers may indeed transmit negative cognitive characteristics to their children which form the basis of a negative self-schema that is activated in response to negative mood-producing stressful events.

DISTAL COGNITIVE REACTIVITY

A proximal paradigm that we have examined at some length, both as a research strategy and as body of data, is the diathesis–stress idea wherein the diathesis is operationalized as an adult who has had an episode of depression and the stress is operationalized in the induction of a negative mood. While there is a considerable body of data for adults, very little data have accrued in the context of distal risk, although a study reported by Timbermont and Braet (2004) has applied this paradigm to children. In particular, groups of children ages 8 to 16 who had, and had not, experienced a previous episode of depression were exposed to a mood induction, and then assessed using an age-appropriate self-referent encoding task. In line with findings in the adult arena, Timbermont and Braet found that remitted children had a negative recall bias after the mood induction.

Summary of Distal Risk Research

Although some distal research has examined cognitive risk without reference to parenting or early experiences (e.g., Timbremont & Braet, 2004), the vast majority of studies do examine these variables in their investigations of cognitive risk. In this regard, the extant data show unquestionably that disrupted interactions with parents pose a risk factor for later depression. Such disruptions may take the form of poor parenting as in lack of care and overcontrol, or may be more malevolent as in the physical, sexual, or emotional abuse of children and adolescents. Theoretical perspectives suggest that the bridge between these parental behaviors and early experiences and later depression in adulthood is cognitive in nature, whether specified as the operations of schemas or the somewhat more inclusive construct of cognitive working models. Thus, the data in this area clearly support the idea that cognitive variables form mediational pathways between troublesome parental–child/adolescent interactions and depression.

SUMMARY

Proximal Cognitive Vulnerability

We began our discussion with a brief review of the diathesis–stress perspective and then examined theory and data relevant to proximal vulnerability. We highlighted the idea of cognitive reactivity in this context, that is, the idea that negative cognitions are reactive to negative events in individuals who are vulnerable to depression. This is particularly important in the examination of proximal vulnerability inasmuch as cognitive depression theories suggest that the proximal cognitive causes of depression are latent until they are activated, and at that point these negative cognitions create a negative spiral that eventuates in depression.

The research evidence solidly supports the critical concepts inherent in cognitive models of depression. For instance, much of the early cognitive research in depression sought to test Beck's (1963, 1967) ideas about the existence and nature of a negative cognitive self-schema. It can safely be concluded that this idea was right in that an abundance of descriptive psychopathology research comparing depressed to nondepressed individuals has found evidence of such schemas across a variety of measures of the construct. But among his earliest writings, Beck also framed this schema in a diathesis–stress context that made clear the idea of cognitive reactivity. Moreover, cognitive reactivity was framed in causal context; the reactive negative schema plays a critical role in the cause of depression. As our review shows, these ideas have received considerable support; across a variety of dependent measures, research has not only found evidence for cognitive reactivity, but also shows that negative cognitive reactions do in fact predict the onset of depressive episodes. Moreover, research focusing on the possession of dysfunctional attitudes and attributional style also supports the ideas of cognitive models.

Distal Cognitive Vulnerability

Proximal research investigates those factors that occur in close proximity to the onset of depression, and thus naturally focus on cognitive
risk in adults. As the support for cognitive models of adult depression
continues to grow, the question becomes one of the origins of these cognitive constructs. Distal risk theory and research addresses this question
in that distal factors are those that occur long before an adult episode
onset and almost surely are developed in childhood and adolescence.
We thus reviewed theories that address cognitive factors in childhood
and adolescence that may be relevant to depression. We also reviewed
research showing that negative early experiences are associated with
negative cognitive factors, that these factors can be detected in high-risk
samples, and that they appear to be activated in much the same way as
adult negative cognitive structures.

This literature is consistent with theories suggesting that aspects of
childhood experiences, such as disrupted attachment with adults and
stressful events, are linked to negative cognitions. More broadly, these
data are consistent with the idea that depressed parents transmit negative cognitive characteristics to their children. That is, negative events
in childhood (including having a depressed parent) may help create the
kinds of cognitive structures that eventually predispose adults to the
experience of depression.

Beyond simply "having" a depressed parent, however, it is important to consider the actual kinds of interactions that may facilitate the
development of negative schemas.

The data suggest in this regard that lack of care seems specifically
linked to cognitive risk. This lack of care can be reflected by neglect in
some cases, or in other cases by excessive criticism or abuse. Moreover,
it seems reasonable to speculate that the long-term effects of negative
events are likely to be particularly virulent when they involve key attachment figures. For example, while neglect may have unpleasant effects
when coming from any important figure, when neglect from significant
others (e.g., parents) is substantial and perhaps chronic, this may produce a particularly negative cognitive self-structure. In the case of neglect
or abuse, the child may develop working models that predispose him or
her to see current or future significant others as neglectful or unreliable,
and may also develop a cognitive representation that views oneself as
unworthy of attention and care (Batagos & Leadbeater, 1995). Similarly,
physically abusive caretakers or significant figures may produce a cogni-

tive model of others as pain producing and not to be trusted, as well as of an unsafe world in general. These children may also develop a cognitive model of themselves as deserving of punishment and pain.

It is worth noting that cognitive structures are not the only neural networks that are developing during these experiences; depending on the developmental level of the child, affective structures are also becoming more differentiated and developing associations to other structures (see Jordan & Cole, 1996). Hence, cognitive self-structures may become closely linked to sadness affective structures through this developmental process. Negative affect thus becomes not only intricately intertwined with unfavorable views of the world and others, but is strongly associated with unfavorable conceptions of the self. If attachment disruptions or other negative events are brief, negative cognitive representations are likely to be limited and more weakly linked to affective networks. On the other hand, if problematic attachment or parenting interactions or negative events are numerous, particularly traumatic, or chronic, then connections between negative self-representations and negative affect may become more extensive and more strongly linked. The soon-to-be-vulnerable-to-depression person thus develops a schema of the self as unlikable and unlovable that is strongly tied to the experience of negative affect. Such networks then becoming available to be brought online when affective structures are activated in the future; when individuals with these cognitive/affective links encounter sadness-producing experiences in the future, they not only experience negative emotions, but will also activate a variety of negative cognitions concerning the self. If this process is indeed the case, then it is easy to see how activation of a negative self-view/negative affect loop can spiral into clinically significant depression.

6

Cognitive Neuroscience Data on Vulnerability

As suggested in Chapter 4, there has been a strong and fruitful surge in interest in the study of emotional processes using cognitive neuroscience techniques. This new research focus, which took hold in the 1990s, can be characterized by a growing attention to topics such as the evolutionary purpose of emotion and the genetic underpinnings of personality traits that might influence individual emotional experience. Additionally, there has been a growing interest in finding neuroscientific corollaries for individual differences in emotion-related processes such as attachment style and temperament. All these issues speak to the question of vulnerability for depression, but many fewer studies have been directly designed to explicitly measure or understand factors of vulnerability. The current outline of research focuses on data that both specifically examines either at-risk populations or depression vulnerability risk factors, and that apply the research tools discussed in Chapter 4 such as electrophysiological, anatomical imaging, and functional imaging methodologies. This organizational scheme recommends that research that applies tools from other areas of neuroscience, including the areas of behavioral genetics, psychopharmacology, and neurochemistry, are more peripherally discussed in the current chapter.

ELECTROPHYSIOLOGICAL RESEARCH

At this point in the development of the field, electrophysiological techniques seem to be the most commonly used methods to directly study depression vulnerability. Reviewed here are example studies from three domains of EEG application: electrophysiological tools that rely on power-spectral analytic techniques for examining patterns of cortical EEG activity, asymmetry, and EEG coherence; a growing body of work that applies polysomnographic techniques to look at patterns of EEG activity during sleep in at-risk populations; and finally a small set of ERP studies that examine cognition-related changes that might be predictive of depression.

Power-Spectral Analytic Research

Davidson and colleagues argue that the two hemispheres of the prefrontal cortex are differentially activated under circumstances that involve decisions on whether to approach or withdraw from a particular object or behavior (Davidson, 2003; Davidson, Jackson, & Kalin, 2000). For example, the prefrontal cortex influences reactions when individuals are faced with uncertainty or when a novel or less comfortable social response is necessary (Davidson, 2003), a circumstance that is also associated with the experience of relatively greater negative emotion and fewer social approach behaviors (Davidson, 1993; Heller et al., 1998). The depression-related pattern of EEG data collected over the prefrontal cortex is specifically a pattern that is indicative of stable asymmetry in frontal lobe activity. Furthermore, this higher asymmetry must be characterized by greater relative left frontal, low frequency or alpha-band frequency EEG activity. Investigations of the relation between frontal brain asymmetry and depression in adults have defined alpha as 9–11 Hz (Schaffer, Davidson, & Saron, 1983), 9–12 Hz (Davidson, Schaffer, & Saron, 1985), or 8–13 Hz (Henriques & Davidson, 1991). It is understood that power in the EEG alpha band is inversely related to cognitive engagement because decreases in alpha tend to be observed when underlying cortical systems engage in active cognitive processing. To understand this general approach, consider Davidson (2003), who tested whether cortical activation is a valid means to guage an individual's sensitivity to emotion elicitation using film clips. In order to detect lateral asymmetries in hemispheric activation, a baseline EEG response was collected as a dependent measure of activation before positive and negative film clips were used to induce a transient valenced mood state. In addition to the EEG measure, participants were asked to rate their emotional experience during the films. Baseline responses were averaged using a within-subjects analysis in order to compare the level of mood change. As predicted, the results showed a positive correlation between patterns of EEG asymmetry and the degree and type of emotion experienced during the films. Participants with EEG activity that is consistent with there being greater cognitive activity in the left hemisphere at baseline rated their experience during the positive films as more affectively positive. In contrast, those participants with a pattern of observed EEG activity that is consistent with a right hemisphere cognitive bias during baseline reported that they experienced negative films as more negative. Davidson (2003) argues that physiological data collected before exposure to the movies indicated a personality bias and effectively predicted participant's reaction to the emotional stimuli. This finding regarding the dominant emotional responses to films and their electrophysiological correlates relates to Davidson's claim (as discussed in some length in Chapter 3) that a specific hemisphere of the prefrontal cortex is activated under circumstances that involve decisions about whether to approach or withdraw from a particular object or behavior (Davidson, 2003; Davidson et al., 2000). In other words, his laterality hypothesis has successfully predicted whether individuals will respond with a valence bias, such as when stronger activation for negative information and more withdrawal-oriented behaviors are observed among individuals who show greater right prefrontal versus left prefrontal activation during baseline measurement. Thus, the next question is, can this affective processing bias be indicative of individuals who are susceptible to depression, but who have not yet developed depression symptoms?

A large cohort of researchers has attempted to answer this question by looking for patterns of EEG asymmetry in at-risk populations (Coan & Allen, 2004). Comparing children with a parental history of depression to a low-risk group of individuals who have mothers and/or fathers most commonly operationalizes vulnerability for depression, in this literature with no history of Axis I psychopathology. Starting with some of the youngest participants that have been studied, several studies have found that infants of depressed mothers do in fact exhibit relative left frontal hypoactivity (e.g., Dawson et al., 1997, 1999, 2006; Field, 2000; Field, Fox, Pickens, & Nawrocki, 1995; Jones, Field, Davalos, & Pickens, 1997; Jones et al., 1998). For example, Dawson et al. (1997) found that at-risk infants showed less left frontal activity than those of nondepressed mothers and that such lower left frontal activity discriminated infants whose mothers were diagnosed with major depression from those with mothers with subthreshold levels of dysphoria. Behaviorally, Dawson and her colleagues have linked left frontal hypoactivity in infants of depressed mothers to observed lower rates of positive affect and increased negative affect during interpersonal interactions (Dawson, Klinger, Panagiotides, Hill, & Spieker, 1992; Dawson et al., 1999). The early age of participants in the Dawson studies lend credibility to the argument that prefrontal cortex patterns of EEG asymmetry might be a good physiological marker of depression risk. However, it is challenging, if not impossible, to know from these reports the degree to which infant frontal EEG asymmetries originate from environmental versus genetic causes. The evidence of similar patterns of prefrontal cortex asymmetry in mothers and infants points to the need for more research on the heritability of prefrontal cortex EEG asymmetry (Coan & Allen, 2003).

Evidence that supports Dawson's findings is provided in the Tomarken, Dichter, Garber, and Simlen (2004) study. Much like in the Dawson work with infants, risk is operationalized via the study of children with depressed mothers; however, in this research the participants were older (between the ages of 12 and 14). Again, high-risk children showed a pattern of left frontal hypoactivity as evidenced by asymmetry in alpha-band power. First, these data suggests that prefrontal cortex asymmetries seen in infants might continue into adolescence. This finding argues that a true longitudinal analysis of asymmetric prefrontal cortex activity would be very helpful. One of the few longitudinal studies that we are aware of (Blackhart, Minnix, & Kline, 2006) that did use prefrontal cortex EEG activity as a predictor found only that left frontal hypoactivity predicted anxiety symptoms in a 1-year follow-up, but not mood measures associated with depression. Tomarken and colleagues (2004) additionally looked at the relationship between prefrontal cortex asymmetry and socioeconomic status (SES). They found that both maternal depression status and SES influence the degree of prefrontal cortex asymmetry, and they found a significant relation between SES and midfrontal asymmetry only in the high-risk group. The authors do not claim to have a clear understanding of the nature of the specific relationship between SES and lateralized prefrontal cortex activity. However, they provide speculation that is consistent with arguments made by Heller and colleagues (Levine, Heller, Mohanty, Herrington, & Miller, 2007) that the elevated levels of daily stressors, poor patterns of health-related behaviors, and other problems associated with low SES clearly increase risk for psychopathology (Johnson, Winett, Meyer, Greenhouse, & Miller, 1999). Their own findings would argue that this socioeconomic risk factor interacts with the genetic and environmental factors associated with paternal pathology, so that we see an overt physiological marker of risk.

Also drawing on data from EEG power spectral measures, Heller and colleagues (1993, 1998) have explored their theory which argues that while the phenomenological experience of emotion is mediated by a frontal lobe valence system, that the perception and expression of emotion is lateralized in the right parietotemporal region of the brain, and that the two systems are functionally interconnected. In support of this two-region model, resting-state EEG studies have revealed that, in addition to prefrontal cortex asymmetries, depression-susceptible individuals show asymmetrical right posterior alpha range activity (Bruder et al., 2005; Bruder, Tenke, Warner, & Weissman, 2007; Hayden et al., 2008). Heller functionally links this posterior EEG pattern to reduced arousal in response to emotionally salient information, which can be manifested as impaired recognition (e.g., Jaeger, Borod, & Peselow, 1986) of emotional cues, such as facial expressions. Thus, impaired recognition of facial affect due to right posterior hypoactivation might help maintain depressive experiences and behaviors as represented by left frontal hypoactivation. For instance, an at-risk person might not register a subtle smile from a neighbor and would thus not experience its positive emotion. Similarly, deficits in the expression of positive facial affect (which is also functionally linked to right parietotemporal brain regions) can induce negative moods in others, leading to degradation of social relationships and even rejection (Segrin, 2001). Consistent with this idea is evidence that infants of depressed mothers exhibit flat affect and may not develop the skills of emotion perception and expression that are needed for social interactions (Field, 1992). Thus, high-risk children with relatively less right parietotemporal activity may be at a disadvantage for perceiving, processing, and responding to positive emotional information, placing them at increased risk for depression.

A growing program of research by Weissman and colleagues (Grillon et al., 2005; Weissman et al., 2005) provides evidence of asymmetric posterior EEG activity in both the children of depressed parents (Bruder et al., 2005) and in high-risk grandchildren (Bruder et al., 2007). Overall, these at-risk groups displayed a parietal alpha asymmetry that might even be a more reliable risk marker than anterior EEG asymmetry. Its presence in high-risk children and grandchildren without a lifetime history of depression supports the hypothesis that an alpha asymmetry indicative of relatively less right than left parietotemporal activity is an endophenotypic marker of vulnerability to depression. A second research team (Hayden et al., 2008) has also found a pattern of relative EEG hypoactivity over left posterior cortical regions that was, in their study, associated with temperamental and cognitive vulnerability to depression (as measured by scales of helplessness and self-reported depression symptoms), in a longitudinal study of 5-, 6-, and 7-year-old children. Interestingly, these researchers only found an effect for posterior asymmetries and did not find a relationship between anterior cortical asymmetry and child temperament, which is consistent with earlier research in this lab (Shankman et al., 2005).

Sleep and Polysomnographic Research

Sleep disruption represents one of the most common symptoms among patients with depression, with something like 80% of patients complaining of this symptom (Reynolds & Kupfer, 1987). In addition to more behaviorally observed kinds of sleep problems, like insomnia, there are also well-documented abnormal sleep events that have been measured using electrophysiological techniques (Armitage, 1995; Armitage & Hoffman, 2001; Berger & Riemann, 1993; Giles, Kupfer, Rush, & Roffwarg, 1998; Knowles & MacLean, 1990; Perlis et al., 1997; Rao et al., 1999). This array includes disturbed sleep maintenance and heightened arousal during sleep, extended Stage 1 sleep duration, a deficit of slow wave sleep (SWS), an earlier onset of the first rapid eye movement (REM) sleep period, changes in delta-band EEG activity, and an increased REM density during REM sleep. However, as with any of the physiological correlates of depression observed, the critical question of interest in this text is if these sleep-related symptoms tell us something about an individual's risk for developing depression.

One of the most extensively documented research programs that has looked at EEG sleep measures and vulnerability for depression is the Munich vulnerability study (see Friess et al., 2008, and Modell, Ising, Holsboer, & Lauer, 2005, for articles that focus on sleep). These researchers, though recognizing that there are many aspects of sleep that are disrupted in currently depressed individuals, make a strong argument that aspects of REM sleep are the most likely sleep component to provide us with a true physiological marker of depression risk. One example of supporting evidence is the finding that premorbid, at-risk participants showed an elevated REM density for the total night as well as for the first sleep cycle compared with control participants. REM density is normally defined via a set of parameters including the number of episodic REMs, bursts of EMG activity (i.e., muscle twitches), and bursts of a stereotypic kind of EEG activity called saw-tooth waves. Aserinsk (1968, 1973) suggested that in sleepers with normal sleep patterns REM density increases across successive REM episodes, approaching its maximum value after at least 7 hours of sleep. Furthermore, Aserinsk and subsequent theorists suggest that REM density might be seen as a measure of sleep satiety, which makes this potential marker intriguing because it implies that for these individuals there are aspects of their sleep that might trigger the body to believe that they have had enough sleep at a point that is too early in the sleep timeline. This work by Aserinski and colleagues has been significantly replicated and extended by additional labs. Giles and colleagues (1998), for example, found that short REM latency and slow wave abnormalities can be seen in the parents and siblings of depressed individuals and that short REM latency is associated with increased risk of major depression. They go on to suggest that sleep abnormalities measured by EEG methods may precede the clinical onset of depression and may be used as a marker for depression vulnerability. Likewise, Modell and colleagues (Friess et al., 2008; Modell, Ising, Holsboer, & Lauer, 2002; Modell et al., 2005) go on to argue that increased REM density (as measured both by total night density and during the first period of REM) satisfy all the major requirements for a valid physiological vulnerability marker for depression because (1) it is seen in patients currently experiencing depression, (2) it is seen in remitted patients, (3) it is present in healthy first-degree relatives of patients, (4) it is stable over time, and (5) it can be used to help predict the onset of the disorder.

ERP Research

The kinds of electrophysiological research on depression vulnerability reviewed so far have focused on more tonic or slow-acting physiological markers, reflecting EEG data collected over minutes or hours. The next section discusses electrophysiological research that attempts to examine risks that might be manifested as an electrophysiological marker that appears during some phasic cognitive response. Engaging in this kind of research blends the cognitive theory discussed elsewhere in this text with neurophysiological data collection methods. This approach for investigating depression vulnerability seems to be the least explored at this point in the development of the field. But it is very likely to see a "growth spurt" as the fields of clinical psychology and cognitive neuroscience become more entwined.

In currently depressed individuals the most consistently studied ERP component is the P300. The P300 component most commonly occurs in response to stimulus events of high *informational salience* (Pritchard, 1981), and its occurrence may be interpreted as signifying the allocation of attentional resources to an identified stimulus (Brandeis et al., 2002; Daffner et al., 2000; Ravden & Polich, 1998), typically as a precursor to more elaborated processing. The most commonly employed methodology for eliciting the P300 waveform is the *oddball task*, in which stimuli are continuously presented in series, the majority of which are highly similar (e.g., all *beeps*) but a small subset of which—the so-called oddballs—are different (e.g., *boops*). The oddball stimulus event, by virtue of its heightened informational salience in context, will typically elicit a robust P300 response, and the presence of an attenuated P300 component is generally indicative of impaired attentional function (Brandeis et al., 2002; Dubal, Pierson, & Jouvent, 2000; Portin et al., 2000). Many studies have examined the P300 component in currently depressed individuals, and they regularly observe an attenuated P300 response in depression across a variety of stimulus types and sensory modalities: auditory tones (e.g., Ancy et al., 1996; Blackwood et al., 1987; Bruder et al., 1995; Murthy, Gangadhar, Janakirmaiah, & Subbakrishna, 1997; Roschke et al., 1996; Torta, Borio, Cicolin, Vighetti, & Ravizza, 1994; Yanai, Fujikawa, Osada, Yamawaki, & Touhouda, 1997), geometric shapes (Chakroun, 1988), alphanumeric characters (Diner, Holcomb, & Dykman, 1985; Pierson et al., 1996), nonsense syllables (Bruder et al., 1991), and photographs (Kayser et al., 2000). Therefore, the most common finding is decreased P300 amplitude in response to neutral, nonaffective stimuli. However, there is also mounting evidence that indicates that depressed individuals show normal or even elevated P300s in response to negative information (Ilardi et al., 2007; Ohira, 1996). Telling a similar story, Cavanagh and Geisler (2006) examined the P300 response of depressed and nondepressed students on an oddball task that presented alternating blocks of rare happy and fearful target expressions interspersed among standard neutral facial stimuli. The authors reported that, compared to the control group, the depressed group showed a reduced mean P300 to happy target faces but not to fearful ones. Therefore, a growing set of data is seen to provide partial evidence for a specificity hypothesis that processing biases are particular to depression-relevant information, such that we see an attenuated P300 for happy or neutral stimuli and a normal or possibly elevated P300 for negative stimuli in currently depressed participants.

As indicated earlier, many fewer studies have examined ERP components related to attention in depression-vulnerable populations. However, abnormal P300 patterns have been found in the few studies that have been published to date (Nikendei, Dengler, Wiedemann, & Pauli, 2005; Perez-Edgar, Fox, Cohn, & Kovacs, 2006; Zhang, Hauser, Conty, Emrich, & Dietrich, 2007). Two of the three vulnerability-P300 studies available continue with the approach of studying individuals who have first-order family members with depression, while the third study chose as their "at-risk" group participants who showed subclinical levels of depression symptoms as measured by the Allgemeine Depressions Skala (Hautzinger & Bailer, 1993). Showing a pattern very consistent with the P300 research done with currently depressed individuals, if at-risk participants are asked to process negatively valent stimuli (Nikendie et al., 2005), then they show an enhanced P300 component, while if they are asked to process affectively neutral stimuli (like large and small letter H's and O's), then at-risk participants show a P300 that is smaller in amplitude than the comparison group (Zhang et al., 2007).

Perez-Edgar and colleagues (2006) took a different approach. They asked participants to do two blocks of a Posner attention task as they collected ERP data. One nice outcome from using the Posner task combined with ERP data collection is that it is thought to allow us to study both early and later attentional mechanisms. ERP studies have indicated that the presentation of a cue seems to engage attention during an early perceptual processing stage (Luck, Heinze, Mangun, & Hillyard, 1990) and this influences the amplitude of early perception-related ERP components (e.g., N1). Specifically it tends to result in increased N1 amplitude on trials with valid cues. In their traditional Posner task block, the participants were asked to detect a target that might appear in one of three locations. On each trial, a precue (a change in color) indicated the probability of the target appearing at that location. Behaviorally there was, as is commonly seen, decreased reaction times in those trials where the target appears at the cued locations (valid cue trials) as compared to trials where the target appeared at the uncued location (invalid cue trials). This is interpreted as a shift of attentional resources to the cued location leading to enhanced processing. In the second block, an affective stressor was added and the participants were told that if their performance during the affective Posner task block was low then they would have to give an embarrassing speech.

The results from these two attention conditions (Perez-Edgar et al., 2006) indicated that at-risk participants do not show an abnormal pattern of selective attention under the neutral affect condition. However, with the introduction of a negative affective stressor, the at-risk participants become far slower in their behavioral responses as compared to the control group. Electrophysiologically, group differences indicate that only later attention-related ERP components differ. Both at-risk and control participants showed the typical N1 amplitude increase on valid trials and this did not change between the neutral and the negative stressor blocks. Where the two groups look most markedly different are during later stages of attentional processing. In both the time range of the P300 and in a time period post 500 milliseconds, often referred to as the slow wave, the control and the at-risk participants differ and they differ most in the affective stressor condition. The authors argue that while the at-risk individuals may perform comparably to participants without a familial history of depression under low-stress conditions, they must deploy greater effortful or strategic processing resources (as reflected by increased ERP amplitudes later in the ERP waveform) and take more time in order to accomplish a similar level of performance. They also speculate that given high enough levels of stress or negative mood state, one may predict that these individuals would no longer be able to engage the necessary compensatory mechanisms to maintain normal performance.

In sum, we have first learned that electrophysiological research can help illuminate neural processes that may underlie homeostatic and cognitive risk factors in individuals who are vulnerable to depression. Predominately by comparing vulnerable individuals to healthy, low-risk individuals with respect to tonic EEG activity (both during wakefulness and sleep), or by looking at the information provided by phasic ERP components, we can shed light on a range of possible variables that are associated with increased risk for depression and that might be seen at a neurophysiological level of analysis.

Anatomical Imaging Research

Based on the range of theories and corresponding neuroanatomical studies of depression discussed in Chapter 4, there is some consensus about what the neuroanatomical regions of interest should be for anatomical imaging studies designed to understand depression vulnerability (see Drevets, Price, & Furey, 2008, for a thorough review of neuroanatomy and neurochemistry research in this area). Specifically, brain regions implicated in the pathology of depression comprise at least two neural systems: (1) a posterior system, including the amygdala, insula, and temporoparietal cortical structures which are utilized in identification of the emotional significance of a stimulus, emotional communication, and automatic regulation of emotional responses; and (2) an anterior system, including the hippocampus, anterior cingulate gyrus, and prefrontal cortex, for the experience and regulation of affective states and subsequent behavior (Heller & Nitschke, 1997; Heller et al., 1998; Kapczinski, Curran, Gray, & Lader, 1994; Kumano et al., 2007; Phillips, Drevets, Rauch, & Lane, 2003). Evidence in support of this notion that either one or both of these neuroanatomical networks should be the focus of depression vulnerability research is both theoretically motivated and includes neuropsychological data such as brain-imaging research that show differences in blood flow or associated measures in these regions in depressed patients (Drevets, 2000, 2008; Drevets et al., 2008; Liotti & Mayberg, 2001). Additionally, in postmortem studies, atrophy or loss of neurons in these regions in patients suffering from depression and anxiety disorders occurs particularly in those patients who have suffered an early childhood trauma (Vythilingam et al., 2002). Therefore, in the current review, the structures of primary focus are the hippocampus, amygdala, cingulate cortex, and prefrontal cortex regions and the primary pattern observed is a decrease in overall volumetric size (Drevets et al., 2008). This does not represent a complete list of structures that have been examined to date, but this review is intended to provide both a summary of the more commonly studied structures and a perspective on how anatomical imaging measures can be effectively utilized to understand depression risk factors. The research to be included in the current section all shares the overarching goal of detecting areas in the brain that are dissociable, either with regards to gross anatomy or with regards to tonic levels of metabolic activity, between individuals who later develop depression and individuals who do not. Of course, these researchers face the same limitations as all the others discussed in the current text, and thus they must rely on various operational definitions of depression risk when selecting participants. However, as we will see, the theorists in this domain often apply new tools to make these very important selections. Specifically, some of the research studies in this particular domain of neuroscience employ neuropharmacological and genetic markers to select their at-risk groups.

Hippocampus

It is widely understood that the hippocampus is involved in many aspects of long-term memory including episodic, declarative, and spatial learning and memory. However, like many structures that are considered part of the classic limbic system, the hippocampus also plays a significant role in emotion processing. One way that the hippocampus plays such a role is through its interactions with the regulation of neuroendocrinatic function tied to the experience and modulation of stress (see Kim & Diamond, 2002, for a thorough review). The hippocampus is a primary target of a class of stress hormones called the corticosteroids. Stress-related hormones play an important role in sculpting the brain because they aid in encoding information that helps us to survive through processes such as long-term potentiation and synaptic selection (Pryce, 2008). One job of the hippocampus is to terminate stress responses and to inhibit and regulate the function of a set of other limbic-related structures including the hypothalamus, pituitary, and adrenal glands (know collectively as the HPA axis). However, during periods of high stress, the presences of high levels of these corticosteroids can have very adverse effects on the hippocampus, causing both morphological changes like cell death or a change in patterns of neurogenesis, and more functional changes such as impediment of synaptic plasticity. All of these outcomes can impede normal learning and memory and they can also impede the hippocampus as it interacts with other limbic structures, such as the amygdala, during emotion regulation functions. Given this memory, stress, and emotion interaction that happens in the hippocampus, the hippocampus is one of the areas in the brain that has been studied in patients with depression, using neuropsychological and neuroimaging studies that consider both memory and learning-related behavioral deficits and structural abnormalities that often accompany depression (Veiel, 1997; Videbech & Ravnkilde, 2004).

Patients with depression have been studied for about 15 years now using MRI techniques to reveal changes in hippocampal volume and density. The results are not always consistent with individual studies. Some volumetric studies have found significantly smaller bilateral volume in depression (MacQueen, Campbell, McEwen, Macdonald, & Young, 2003; McEwen & Magarinos, 2001; Sheline et al., 1996). Others have found unilateral deficits in volume (Bremner et al., 2000; Mervaala et al., 2000). Still other studies have failed to find any differences between depressed and nondepressed participants in hippocampal volume (Rusch, Abercrombie, Oakes, Schaefer, & Davidson, 2001; von Gunten, Fox,

Cipolotti, & Ron, 2000). However, in a recent meta-analysis (Videbech & Ravnkilde, 2004), it was concluded that depressed patients do show consistently smaller hippocampal volume than nondepressed comparison groups and that these differences occur bilaterally. If the research regarding the impact of stress on hippocampal cell vitality is correct, then it would seem appropriate to assume that reductions of hippocampal volume is an outcome of depression and not a preexisting condition that acts as a risk factor. Nonetheless, a small number of researchers have specifically looked to see if smaller hippocampal volume might precede the onset of depression.

One study that was designed to address this question was by Vythilingam and colleagues (2002). This was not a prospective study. Instead, they compared 32 participants with current depression who had either experienced childhood trauma (in the form of prepubertal sexual or physical abuse; 21) or who had not (11). The assumption of course was that the stress caused by the abuse had an adverse effect on hippocampal volume and that this diminishment of normal hippocampal volume preceded the onset of depression. Consistent with their hypotheses, they found that only the patients who had experienced abuse showed a reduced hippocampal volume. This observed correlation was in part a way to explain some of the variability in the early MRI literature, discussed above, on depression and hippocampal volume. They also argue that reduced hippocampal size might be particularly likely in patients who have a treatment-resistant and/or severe depression (Mervaala et al., 2000). One big problem with using this Vythilingam et al. study to argue that hippocampal volume creates greater risk for depression is that they did not have the desired control group of participants who had experienced abuse, but who had not developed depression.

A second effort to address our central question, which was carried out by Frodl and colleagues (2002), compared first-episode depression patients to healthy controls. This approach clearly helps avoid looking at hippocampal differences that might best be explained as resulting from the stress and emotional disturbances that one experiences during prolonged or repeated acute depressive episodes. This study was also interesting in that the researchers collected a sufficient sample of male and female participants so that gender analyses were appropriate. For the male participants, the first-episode patients had a reduced unilateral (left) hippocampal grey-matter volume and both genders showed significantly lesser white-matter volume in the depressed participants as compared to the controls. One possible explanation that the authors offer for their gender findings might be the neuroprotective effects of estrogen, which has been seen in both animal models and human studies, while in contrast testosterone may actually exacerbate vulnerability to the neurotoxic effects of the corticosteroids. This hypothesis seems to lead to the idea that the impact of high stress on hippocampal tissue might act as a greater risk factor for males than for females.

A third approach that has been taken to determine if hippocampal size might constitute a risk factor for psychopathology is to compare monozygotic twins who are discordant for stress-related experiences that make them at risk for developing depression (de Geus et al., 2007; Gilbertson et al., 2002). This approach has the potential to be very helpful because it allows for good control over the impact of genetic variability, which might mitigate the stress–hippocampal change–depression timeline that is being suggested. The twin study that most specifically focused on the development of depression (as compared to the Gilbertson et al. work that looked at the development of PTSD, but speaks to issues important for affective disorders more generally) compared three sets of monozygotic twins. This study (de Geus et al., 2007) compared hippocampal volume for seven high-risk pairs of twins who had concordant environmental and interpersonal risk for depression, 15 low-risk pairs of twins who had concordant risk for depression, and 10 twin pairs who were discordant in their depression risk. Risk was estimated based on longitudinal survey data on anxiety, depression, neuroticism, and somatic anxiety (Boomsma et al., 2000). For the two concordant pairs of twins there was no difference in hippocampal volume either between each pair of twins, or in comparing the high- and low-risk groups. This finding is important to note because it suggests that when we compare across these genetically variable samples, we do not see direct evidence of risk in hippocampal volume. However, consistent with study predictions, in comparing the individuals in the discordant twin pairs, hippocampal volume does differ, and the high-risk twin showed significantly smaller hippocampal volume. Thus, the authors draw the strong conclusion that the genetic and environmental etiology of mood disorder may differ and that damage to the hippocampal region may be specific to the environmentally driven etiology of depression.

Amygdala

The amygdala has become increasingly of interest to researchers trying to understand depression for many good reasons. It makes sense to look at the anatomy and function of the amygdala given the theory and data that we just reviewed on hippocampal functioning in depression. The hippocampus and amygdala are highly interconnected physiologically and, as discussed earlier, the hippocampus acts as a kind of regulator for amygdalar function. Additionally, there is a growing imaging literature looking at mood regulation that implicates the amygdala as important. As is discussed in the functional imaging section, the amygdala seems to be overresponsive to negative stimuli in depression (Drevets et al., 2002), and insufficiently regulated by prefrontal cortex structures (Drevets et al., 1997; Ito et al., 1996; Pascual-Leone, Rubio, Pallardo, & Catala, 1996). Finally, alteration in the genes that influence the serotonergic system is associated with augmented amygdala response to emotional stimuli. A great deal of work from many domains has focused on the role of serotonin in the development of depression. Serotonin has been implicated in a number of processes in brain development and synaptic plasticity in part through this hippocampal–amygdalar circuit and low levels of serotonin have been associated with susceptibility to mood regulation problems seen in depression and anxiety (Frodl, Moller, & Meisenzahl, 2008; Meltzer et al., 1998). Furthermore, selective serotonin reuptake inhibitors (SSRIs) have proven effective in the treatment of many affective disorders (Goodnick & Goldstein, 1998). This evidence has led to the examination of the role of the genes that influence this serotonergic system.

The polymorphism that has been the focus of most research on the serotonergic system is an insertion/deletion polymorphism (*5-HTTLPR*), which is characterized by both long and short allele-type variants (Lesch et al., 1996). For example, previous studies have reported that individuals with a deletion polymorphism that results in one or two short alleles in this region who experience negative life stress are at greater risk for depression than individuals with two long alleles (Caspi et al., 2003; Kendler, Kuhn, Vittum, Prescott, & Riley, 2005). Carriers of the short *5-HTTLPR* allele may be less efficient in regulating serotonin reuptake at the presynaptic neuron, with consequences for signaling and the communication with postsynatptic receptors, compared to carriers of the long allele. Given serotonin's role in regulating neural circuits that subsume the processing of emotion information, such differences may explain why short *5-HTTLPR* allele carriers are more likely to respond to life stress with depressive reactions. Thus, research has indicated a number of potential physiological mechanisms by which the *5-HTTLPR* may influence the serotonergic system and ultimately increase the likelihood of depression (Frodl et al., 2008; Owens & Nemeroff, 1994), but for this discussion we focus on the relationship between *5-HTTLPR* and altered HPA axis function. We include a review of research that examines the role that this polymorphism might play in biased attention in Chapter 8.

Jabbi et al. (2007) observed an increase in HPA axis excitability in response to stress in females expressing a version of the short *5-HTTLPR* allele. Similar abnormalities in HPA axis responses have been observed in 5-HTT knockout mice (Tjurmina, Armando, Saavedra, Goldstein, & Murphy, 2002). Hariri et al. (2002) examined *5-HTTLPR*'s relationship to the amygdala's response to fearful stimuli. While the amygdala is more typically associated with the expression of fear and anxiety, it is plausible that the short *5-HTTLPR* allele could potentially affect one's perception of stressful life events. These differing perceptions of stressful life events could explain why some individuals develop major depression in response to stressful life events, while other individuals are seemingly unaffected by such events. Thus further research looking at the role that this *5-HTTLPR* polymorphism plays could provide better insight into how functioning in the amygdala and other related subcortical structures might act as a physiological risk factor for depression.

In addition to considering amygdalar activity levels, as mediated by serotonin, anatomical researchers have also looked at overall amygdala volume as a possible contributing factor, or at least a part of a causal chain of phenomena that might increase depression risk (see Andersen & Teicher, 2008, for a review). As with consideration of hippocampal volume, it makes sense to look at the volumetric size of the amygdala because it too can be diminished over time due to the toxic effects of high levels of corticosteroids. Volumetric differences between currently depressed and never depressed individuals at first glance seems to be somewhat less clear than is the case for the hippocampus, but as reviewed in a meta-analysis by Hamilton, Siemer, and Gotlib (2008), the differences in amygdala size might be real, but may be mitigated or even reversed via neurotrophic processes caused by antidepressant medications. Thus, like with the hippocampus, the amygdala seems to be smaller in volume in currently depressed individuals if they are not being treated with antidepressants. Although this observed relationship between medication status and amygdala volume is certainly suggestive, trying to find research that examines amygdalar volume in individuals who are at risk, but who have not developed depression yet, is difficult. A few studies have assessed participants who are newly diagnosed

(Kronenberg et al., 2009; van Eijndhoven et al., 2009), but these studies provide inconsistent findings, with the Kronenberg et al., study showing smaller amygdala size in depressed participants and the van Eijndhoven et al., work reporting enlarged amygdalar volume in early depression. Furthermore, these studies are not ideal for trying to look at pre-onset risk factors because the participants are severe enough to warrant diagnosis and treatment, and there are no anatomical imaging studies that we are aware of that allow us to look at the desired sample of at-risk participants. However, as we will see in the functional imaging section, the desired study has been conducted assessing amygdalar functioning in children with a family history of depression (Monk et al., 2008).

Cingulate Cortex

The cingulate cortex forms a large region that is just superior to the corpus callosum and represents the most medial portion of the cerebral cortexes. This region has numerous projections into motor systems and so one function associated with the area is motor control and planning, but functional studies have shown that this region contributes to a number of other brain functions (see Devinsky, Morrell, & Vogt, 1995, for a review of cingulate functional anatomy). Therefore, the region is further subdivided into "affective" and "cognitive" systems. The structures that play a role in emotion processes have extensive connections with the prefrontal cortex, hypothalamus, thalamus, amygdala, hippocampus, and entorhinal cortex, and parts of it project to autonomic brainstem motor nuclei. In addition to regulating more subcortical endocrinatic functions, it is involved in conditioned emotional learning, expressions of internal states, assessments of internal motivational states, and assigning emotional valence to internal and environmental stimuli. Humans with lesions including the cingulate cortex can show impaired emotional processing in the absence of significant cognitive impairment. Thus, given its significant role in emotion processing, the cingulate has been of great interest to researchers studying affective disorders such as depression.

A meta-analysis of anatomical imaging work (both using voxel-based morphometry, such as MRI, and postmortem techniques) on cingulate volume in patients with mood disorders confirms this hypothesis that structural abnormalities in cingulate anatomy are correlated with the experience of depression (Hajek, Kozeny, Kopecek, Alda, & Hoschl, 2008). The authors argue that the research in this particular domain has been fortunate to be remarkably consistent methodologically. In part because of this uniformity in methodology, the authors were able to look beyond the simple comparison of depressed versus never depressed participants and ask questions of interest in the domain of depression vulnerability. Specifically, they were able to subdivide their depressed participants into individuals who had a family history of mood disorders from those with no family history. Their meta-analysis included a total of eight studies with 210 patients (99 with bipolar disorder and 111 with unipolar depression). The conclusions from this study do much to speak to the question of vulnerability, even though it was designed to be a meta-analysis of studies examining currently depressed individuals. First, there was a general finding of reduced cingulate volume in patients with depression. But this correlation seemed to be limited to depressed participants who also had a family history of depression. Thus the authors conclude that this points to the possibility of a genetically instantiated risk. Additionally, the authors argue that differences in cingulate volume are not a secondary result of depression experience in that cingulate volume was not correlated with the number of depressive episodes experienced or length of depressive episodes. Furthermore, in the two more longitudinal studies of depression, unlike hippocampal volume, cingulate size did not decrease over time. Therefore, the authors conclude that cingulate volume might represent a vulnerability marker and not a scarring effect generated by depression experience.

Following up on this kind of retrospective approach to understanding the role that cingulate morphology might play in depression risk is work by Boes, McCormick, Coryell, and Nopoulos (2008) who provide the only prospective study of cingulate structure and vulnerability that we have found. Boes and colleagues considered many important characteristics of a group of 112 healthy children (ages 7 to 17) including cingulate volume, mood symptomatology, and family history of depression. This research lends partial support to the argument that cingulate volume may be a neuronantomical marker for depression risk. In the female half of the child sample, there was no clear relationship between the degree of depression symptoms, family depression history, and cingulate size. The authors suggest that this aspect of their findings may reflect sampling error, in that they observed unexpectedly low levels of depression symptoms in their female sample. However, in the male children sampled, there was the expected relationship. First, there was a significant correlation between cingulate volume and depression symptoms such that higher mood disturbance was correlated with smaller cingulate volume. Additionally, this correlation was only observed in the portion of the sample who would be considered at risk because of a history of depression in first-order relatives. The authors of this work point out that they cannot rule out the possibility that some of their participants were experiencing undiagnosed juvenile depression because no clinical interview was performed. However, this research does represent an attempt to extend this cingulate–depression relationship beyond the study of individuals with the current pathological conditions, thus providing further support for arguments that smaller cingulate volume might be a genetically mediated marker for depression risk.

Prefrontal Cortex

A common finding is alterations in volume and neurophysiological activity in the medial prefrontal cortex and related areas in the orbital prefrontal cortex in patients with recurrent depression (Drevets et al., 2008). These prefrontal regions are also part of a larger system of cortical areas that include the cingulate cortex, along with areas in the right parietal regions, and the hippocampal formation, which has been implicated in emotional self-reference and emotional communication. Thus, dysfunctions involving prefrontal cortex regions not only induce disturbances in general emotional behavior because of disrupted modulation of the hypothalamus and brainstem, which leads to disturbances in more autonomic emotion-related physiological regulation, but are also thought to effect more complex cognitive aspects of emotion processing. For example, prefrontal damage can lead to a disruption in the interpretation of more subtle emotional stimuli or affective planning that occur in social circumstances (see Davidson, Pizzagalli, Nitschke, & Putnam, 2002, for a review). Therefore, given the functional significance of the prefrontal cortex, it is likely that, like with the other brain regions discussed, we might expect to see that a smaller volumetric size in prefrontal cortex regions may precede and contribute to the onset of depression. It should be noted that in a related literature, particularly focused on older at-risk patients, the precursor for depression may be characterized by a different manifestation of prefrontal hypoactivity and this is a phenomena called "white-matter hyperintensity" which is not a decrease in overall volume but an increase in MRI-measured markers of tissue damage reflecting, primarily, vascular disease (Oda et al., 2003).

Evidence consistent with this kind of prediction comes from a few different sources (Koenigs et al., 2008; Kumano et al., 2007; Ma et al., 2007; Taki et al., 2005). One source that relies on a different methodology than discussed so far in this chapter is a very interesting comparative study by Leussis and Andersen (2008). We have not spent much time talking about animal model-based research, but this study lends itself nicely to the current discussion because it specifically addresses prefrontal cortex anatomy and its relationship to depression vulnerability, response to environmental stressors, and depression-related symptom patterns. The general conclusion of the study comparing male and female rats is that when the animals are exposed to social stressors (i.e., social isolation) during a period that represents the adolescent period of development, then we see some interesting physiological and behavioral ramifications. Behaviorally, the depression symptoms that were manifested more frequently by stressed rats were a pattern of more frequent and more rapid onset of periods of immobility during a stressful situation (such as a forced swim) combined with evidence of more learned helplessness. Physiologically, the experience of stress during the rat's adolescent period lead to a regionally specific decline, in the prefrontal cortex, for protein types (e.g., spinophillin and synaptophysin) that are generally thought to allow for the development of normal synaptic transmission (Becher et al., 1999; Feng et al., 2000). Additionally these researchers begin to provide some indication about why some depressed participants develop one pattern of cortical abnormality (such as a reduction in more subcortical limbic regions like the hippocampus) while others may have more cortical disruptions. In comparing across studies, they found that the age of stress exposure was important for determining what pattern of cortical decline was observed, with younger stress exposure leading to more hippocampal disruption (Andersen & Teicher, 2004) and later exposure to stress, during the rat's adolescence, leading to greater disruption in cortical development (Leussis & Andersen, 2008).

However, the story regarding the prefrontal cortex is likely more complex than the reframe that has become the pattern in this literature, the idea that smaller, less developed anatomy increases depression risk. We know that the prefrontal cortexes are best understood as a complex network of structures that do not behave in a holistic fashion (see Fuster, 1997, 2001). Consistent with this general consensus, recent research has argued that prefrontal regions may contribute differently to the onset of depression. Koenigs and colleagues (2008) found opposite effects with regards to the onset of depression symptoms when they compared patients who had lesions to the ventromedial and dorsal regions of the prefrontal cortex. In the ventromedial patient sample, significantly lower depression symptoms were observed when compared to patients with damage involving other areas of the brain or patients with no brain damage. In addition, one patient with a premorbid history of depression experienced a dramatic reduction of depressive symptoms, particularly the cognitive/affective symptoms, after bilateral ventromedial damage. In contrast, with patients with dorsal prefrontal damage, greater depression symptom severity was observed and these patients were more likely to have symptom severity high enough to warrant diagnose with major depression. The authors point to confirmatory work using transcranial magnetic stimulation and other methods of brain stimulation, which has shown that an antidepressant effect can result from either stimulation of dorsolateral regions (Avery et al., 2006; Berman et al., 2000) or the inhibition of ventromedial areas (Mayberg et al., 2005). Even though the Koenigs et al. study does not specifically address an at-risk group, it does suggest that future research examining anatomical distinctions in prefrontal cortex between vulnerable and less vulnerable participants would need to be cognizant that more fine-grain anatomical analysis might be critical to seeing a clear pattern of results.

In summary, it is clear that like with all the electrophysiological methods, more research using converging definitions of depression vulnerability is warranted. It is also clear that a general pattern is emerging that allows for reasonably clear a priori predictions. Genetic factors and environmental stressors can both result in a hypogenesis or degeneration of critical limbic system structures. Following this structural disruption we would then expect to see a disruption of normal neuronal functioning that underlies the general depression symptomatology. However, as we move on to the consideration of functional imaging studies, one can not always predict that structural reductions will result in neuronal hypoactivity because of the dual excitatory and inhibitory nature of normal neuronal functioning. So during the next section the goal is to determine what kinds of region-specific neuronal functioning difference can be seen in patients who are at risk for depression.

Functional Imaging Research

When considering the growing body of research that applies functional imaging tools for the general purpose of understanding the functional anatomy of depression, three observations emerge. First, the portion of the literature that looks at current depression is rather large, which reflects the utility of applying functional imaging tools to address the range of cognitive processes that might be affected in depression or mood-disordered populations (Davidson & Irwin, 1999; Drevets, 1998; Haldane et al., 2008; Koenigs & Grafman, 2009; Liotti & Mayberg, 2001; Phan, Wager, Taylor, & Liberzon, 2004). More importantly, a second summative observation that can be made is that there is a strong degree of convergence across cognitive neuroscience methods, which suggests that the research community is probably on the "right track." For example, the anatomical imaging literature suggests that specific brain regions (i.e., the amygdala, hippocampal formation, prefrontal cortex, and cingulate regions) should be foci of functional distinctions between depressed and nondepressed participants. Consistent with this prediction, this network of limbic structures is implicated as areas of functional differences in mood-disordered participants (Haldane & Franguo, 2008; Phan et al., 2004). Going back to the EEG and ERP work reviewed, the suggestion would be that certain tasks should be discriminatory, specifically, during exposure to stressful or affectively charged stimuli, or when selective attention, categorization, and encoding resources are employed. It is predicted that these two broad cognitive domains are modulated by depression and, again, the fMRI data typically concurs (Davidson & Irwin, 1999; Haldane & Franguo, 2008; Liotti & Mayberg, 2001). The final observation that might be made is that the number of studies that use functional imaging to study initial depression risk are surprisingly low. One might expect, given the large volume of research looking at current depression, that there would a lot to learn about depression vulnerability as well, but this just has not proven to be the case to date. We can supplement this smaller portion of research by considering work looking at risk for depression relapse in remitted depressed patients (Drevets et al., 1992; Gemar, Segal, Mayberg, Goldapple, & Carney, 2007; Hooley et al., 2009; Ramel et al., 2007; Smith et al., 2002). Nonetheless, it seems clear that given the general flexibility, utility, and accessibility of functional imaging methods, this is an area of research that must clearly grow substantially if we wish to better understand depression vulnerability.

Impact of Stress and Mood on Functional Activity

The bulk of research that has directly addressed the domain of depression vulnerability using functional imaging falls into this first cognitive processing category (Drevets et al., 1992; Gemar et al., 2007; Harvey, Pruessner, Czechowska, & Lepage, 2007; Hooley et al., 2009; Mak, Hu, Zhang, Xiao, & Lee, 2009; Pezawas et al., 2005; Smith et al., 2002;

Smith, Henson, Dolan, & Rugg, 2004). In general, these studies take the approach of comparing functional scans taken under two or three conditions, either during a period of high stress or negative emotion induction, under a period of positive emotion, and finally during a period of neutral affect or low stress. In some respects, this approach mimics the methodological goals of the EEG- power spectral work discussed earlier that looked at lateralized differences in prefrontal cortex activity in response to emotional stimuli (Davidson, 2003; Davidson et al., 2000). The parallel goal here is to look at general levels of neuronal metabolic activity in key limbic areas when at-risk participants are exposed to emotion-invoking situations.

Hooley and colleagues (2009) provide an example of this approach that exemplifies this category of research in part because the authors were careful to examine most of the ROIs (regions of interest) that have been the focus of the theoretical models reviewed here. In their study they compared fully remitted participants to never depressed participants as they were exposed to three different affective conditions that seem to have very good "face validity." The researchers contacted, via telephone, the mothers of the study participants and asked them to make specific comments about their children that were either critical or praising in their affective value. Mothers chose the content of each criticizing or praising comment. Thus they were likely to be both specific and very personal. For control purposes the researchers ensured that each comment lasted 30 seconds and had a fairly systematic structure (e.g., "Stephanie, one thing that really bothers me about you is … " or "Stephanie, one thing I really like about you is … "). In addition to providing critical and praising comments, mothers were also asked to provide neutral comments that were general and not about their own child.

Behaviorally (as reflected by reported mood change on the Positive Affect Negative Affect Schedule) these two emotional challenge conditions (praise vs. criticism) caused equal mood change in the remitted and comparison groups. Furthermore, both caused the expected mood change, with praise causing an elevation in mood and criticism causing a more negative mood state. The neuroimaging data from the remitted group were compared directly with the data from the control group. Levels of activation in the amygdala were similar in both groups when they heard praise or neutral comments. However, when the remitted participants heard criticism (compared with resting baseline), they showed significantly greater blood-oxygen-level-dependent (BOLD) activation than the controls within the amygdala. Thus, shifts in amygdala activation are only seen for negative affective stimuli and the pattern of results suggests hyperactivity in the amygdala during a negative experience. For the cortical regions the group differences were more affectively general. The remitted participants showed significantly less BOLD activation than the controls in both the prefrontal cortex and the anterior cingulate gyrus in all three affective conditions. When the remitted participants simply heard their mothers talk, even when the topic was very impersonal, such as a comment about the weather, this led to hypoactivation of the prefrontal cortex and the cingulate gyrus in the remitted participants as compared to the participants who were less vulnerable to depression.

Assuming that future researchers replicate the variety of data observed by Hooley and colleagues (2009), these findings are very informative. First, they suggest that risk factors for depression may be observable using functional imaging methods even when overt behavioral responses suggest that the at-risk group is no different in their experience than a low-risk group. Neurophysiologically, there are two possibly dissociable, possibly interrelated patterns that seem to emerge. First there seems to be higher amygdala activation in response to negative or stressful stimuli in at-risk individuals (Bremner et al., 2003; Drevets et al., 1992; Hooley et al., 2009). This finding has also been seen in both rhesus monkey models of affective disorder (Kalin et al., 2008) and in humans (see Brown & Hariri, 2006, for a review), where individuals who exhibit the short allele type of a functional polymorphism (*5-HTTLPR*) within the serotonin transporter gene show increased amygdala reactivity when they are exposed to aversive or stressful stimuli.

The second neurophysiological pattern that emerges is that in conditions of emotional significance (possibly regardless of the specific emotional content) hypoactivity of cortical regions are observed in at-risk participants. This was found by Holley and colleagues (2009) and by researchers such as Gemar et al. (2007) and Mak and colleagues (2009). In a complimentary finding Harvey et al. (2007) found prefrontal hyperactivity in a positive picture condition in a sample of nonclinical participants experiencing anhedonia. Harvey and colleagues argued that this increase in prefrontal activity in response to the positive stimulus represents an effortful focus on positive cues, which might act to reduce their negative mood state. Thus, a problem that might emerge is that in individuals who are more vulnerable to depression they may fail to engage in effortful, prefrontally mediated, compensatory strategies that might help to repair mood (Keedwell, Andrew, Williams, Brammer, & Phillips, 2005).

Selective Attention and Memory Functions

Given the focus on attention and memory changes as symptoms of depression, it is surprising that more research has not been done to look at these cognitive processes using functional imaging in at-risk samples. The research discussed above also suggests that this approach of studying attention and memory functions in depression-vulnerable individuals would be fruitful given that the brain structures effected during tonic negative mood induced by affective stressors specifically influence the regions that support these two important cognitive functions. There were only four examples of this kind of work that we could find to date, three focusing on categorization and memory (Chan, Harmer, Goodwin, & Norbury, 2008; Ramel et al., 2007; Wolfensberger et al., 2008) and one examining selective attention using an emotional Stroop paradigm (Mannie et al., 2008). The first memory study to be discussed is a study of remitted and never depressed individuals published by Ramel and colleagues (2007), the second memory study examined monozygotic twins who were concordant or discordant for depression risk (Wolfenberger et al., 2008), and the third memory study looked at risk by comparing nondepressed participants that are high and low in neuroticism (Chan et al., 2008). The sole selective attention study utilized two samples of never depressed participants, one group who had a familial history of major depression while the low-risk group had no family history of psychological disorder (Mannie et al., 2008).

All three memory studies reviewed looked at encoding and recall of emotionally valanced words. The work by Ramel and colleagues (2007) more specifically focused on patterns of encoding for negative and positive self-referent words using a sad mood induction paradigm. Consistent with cognitive research in this domain, these researchers predicted that the evaluation and recall of negative self-descriptive words would be especially salient for individuals with a history of depression during a transient mood challenge. The expected mechanism for this effect was predicted to be activation of a amygdala-modulated, cognitive-affective network that contributes to deeper encoding of negative self-referent words and, thus, to enhanced retrieval of these words for remitted participants compared with never depressed individuals. Behaviorally, the authors report no group difference in recall pattern for negative self-referent words, though the remitted depressed were proportionally less likely to recall positive self-referent words. Prior to mood induction there were no differences in amygdala activity across group or valence conditions, and no relationship between amygdala activity and recall rate. After mood induction, however, amygdala response to negative versus positive words predicted proportionate negative self-referent recall in remitted participants but not in the control group. Furthermore, this significant correlation between amygdala activity and recall rate was only found for negative self-referent words and not for any other word condition. The results from this study are a bit subtler than others reported in that a general increase in amygdala activity was not observed in the remitted group, nor were negative self-referent words preferentially recalled. But this research does provide a more subtle insight into neurocognitive mechanisms in that it suggests that the amygdala is preferentially involved in negative self-referent word encoding and recall only when the at-risk individual is feeling sad. Thus, this gives us a more precise understanding of at least one role that the amygdala may play in depression-vulnerable individuals.

Wolfensberger et al. (2008) have a more expanded anatomical focus with their work in that their ROIs also focused in the cerebral cortex, specifically in prefrontal regions and the medial temporal lobe. As with Ramel and colleagues, the participants in this study were scanned as they first classified and encoded words varying in emotional valence, and then in a second scan period recalled these words (though Wolfensberger et al. did not look at the variable of self-reference). Also, as with the study with remitted depressed participants, behavioral data were not very effective at discriminating between groups. The neurophysiological data again proved to be more sensitive to vulnerability variables in that they found clear evidence that brain activation during encoding and retrieval of emotional stimuli is indeed influenced by both genetic and environmental risk factors. During encoding, the researchers found increased activity in prefrontal cortex regions in concordant high-risk twins as compared to the concordant low-risk twins across all word types. Discordant twin pairs did not show this difference. During recognition the same elevation in prefrontal activity was found in high-risk twins as compared to low-risk participants, this time in both discordant and concordant pairs, but this elevation in activity was only observed for negative words. Previous research in the more mainstream cognitive neuroscience literature suggests that greater activation is found in these same prefrontal regions for "remembered" as compared to "forgotten" words (Baker, Sanders, Maccotta, & Buckner, 2001). The results could be seen to argue that high-risk participants may need to work harder to categorize emotional words. Additionally, this increased effort and elaboration preferentially impacts negative stimuli. Outside the cerebral cortex additional differential effects of negative words with the low- and high-risk participants were found, specifically during encoding. Consistent with the Ramel et al. (2007) study, high-risk individual twins showed greater amygdala activity during the processing and encoding of negative words as compared to their low-risk cotwins.

Finally, Chan and colleagues (2008) expand the list of ROIs even further and consider the contribution that more parietal cortical regions might play in affective memory encoding. High-risk participants in this study was operationally defined as never depressed individuals who scored high in neuroticism on the Eysenck Personality Questionnaire (Eysenck, Eysenck, & Barrett, 1985). The researchers argue that there is a good deal of evidence to suggest that high levels of neuroticism is a strong predictor of future depression (Kendler, Gardner, & Prescott, 2002; Kendler, Gatz, Gardner, & Pederson, 2006). Again, encoding and retrieval data did not differ across either risk group or word valence. However, the neurophysiological data illustrates that high risk is associated with greater activity in the right parietal cortex in high-risk rather than low-risk participants, specifically during the categorization and encoding of negative words. The risk factor of neuroticism was also found to be correlated with increased activity in the anterior cingulate during the categorization of negative possibly self-referent words and reduced activity within this same area during the retrieval of these negative words, and this correlation is specifically driven by the high-risk participants.

All of the memory studies reviewed here are consistent with early work reviewed in that they find that depression risk seems to impact limbic processing in a way that is more easily observed when looking at neurophysiological data than with looking at behavioral data alone. But unlike the earlier section covering functional imaging research looking at more tonic mood effects, the results here are quite complex and nuanced. For example, in the Wolfensberger (2008) study the comparison of risk in concordant versus discordant twins suggests that genetic versus more environmental risk factors likely influence different parts of the limbic network. Furthermore, it is clear that a very wide range of risk variables and brain regions need to be more systematically studied. Therefore, before we can extract any clear conclusions about risk from functional imaging work on memory, more work needs to be done.

In order to study attention-related processes, Stroop tasks have been used during functional imaging with currently depressed participants in the literature (George et al., 1997; Wagner et al., 2006). Like with research from the traditional cognitive neuroscience domain (Whalen et al., 1998), the primary region of focus for most functional imaging is the cingulate cortex. The general finding that would be expected in healthy, normally functioning individuals would be that during the perception of emotion-laden words, cingulate activity should increase, reflecting an increase in attention resources when the distracting emotional message might interfere with the primary task, such as counting the number of words presented (Compton et al., 2003). Mannie and colleagues (2008) continued with this approach in their study of emotion-counting Stroop words in high-risk versus low-risk young adults. For this study risk is, again, defined by familial history of depression. The researchers' a priori prediction was that participants with high depression risk would show lower activation of critical anterior cingulate regions during the counting of physically (*accident*) or socially (*inferior*) threatening words. Again, no behavioral differences were found for any of the variables of study. Consistent with earlier work, the low-risk participants showed significantly more cingulate activity in the negative and positive Stroop blocks as compared to the block of neutral words. In contrast, the high-risk participants, despite their equal behavioral performance, showed no modulation in cingulate activity for either negative or positive words. This result was taken to suggest that, despite the fact that these at-risk individuals have never experienced depression, they are still less able to inhibit the emotional content of the words and are, likewise, less efficient at detecting key differences in the emotional content of environmental input.

In summary, the results from all of these functional imaging studies indicate that abnormalities in the neural response to emotional stimuli, in a range of limbic system structures, can exist independently of the presence of behavioral evidence or acute dysphoria. Furthermore, they appear to be present in individuals who are at risk of depression, but who have never experienced a depressive episode. Given the striking findings from these few studies, it seems critical for more researchers to use functional imaging methods to look at the integration of emotional and cognitive information via the application of online cognitive tasks. Deficits in this sort of cognitive processing could result in difficulties in many domains including during social interactions and the internal integration of past experience into an internal self-schema. Thus, the sensitive study of relatively simple cognitive mechanisms allowed for by functional imaging methods could provide us with a clearer picture about how increased risk of depression can be expressed.

SUMMARY

We know a good deal about how the brains of currently depressed and nondepressed individuals tend to differ. To the extent that this research is applicable to depression risk, investigators have tended to make inferences on the basis of studies of currently depressed individuals. As we noted in Chapter 4, however, such inferences run the risk of being unable to differentiate processes that precede the disorder and those that arise either concomitantly with or are caused by the disorder. It is thus clear that much more research needs to be done utilizing cognitive neuroscience methods to study depression vulnerability. But as we have reviewed here, an empirical start has been made on understanding the neuroscience of vulnerability.

The prefrontal cortex is the area that has been the focus of the most converging cognitive neuroscience: vulnerability research. Specifically, an at-risk person seems to have a prefrontal cortex that is generally hypoactive or preferentially hypoactive over the left hemisphere. The prefrontal cortex is important because this structure contributes to the control and allocation of selective attention, executive functions, mood, and some aspects of memory encoding, and disruption of these cognitive functions have been seen in at-risk individuals.

There are also converging data to point to the cingulate as a region that should inspire future research regarding risk for depression. The P300 ERP component can be abnormal in at-risk participants and many ERP researchers have seen the cingulate as an important source for at least one of the components in the P300 family. There is also the enticing, though small, bit of evidence discussed here that suggests that the cingulate cortex might be smaller in volume in individuals (particularly men) who are at risk for depression. Given the role that the cingulate cortex plays in a range of cognitive functions that are central to depression symptomatology, including functions such as reward anticipation, decision making, motivation, and emotion, more research needs to be done to confirm whether cingulate-centered abnormalities precede depression onset.

A classic limbic system structure that has been examined using cognitive neuroscience tools is the amygdala. The anatomical imaging data looking at amygdala size in at-risk individuals is inconclusive, although the neurochemical research (particularly the genetics research examining the serotonergic system) and fMRI studies converge to suggest that the amygdala seems to be either hyperactive or hyperresponsive to certain kinds of stimuli in individuals who are at risk. Given that the human amygdala is beginning to be understood as a complex, functionally subdivided structure involved in emotion processing, learning, memory, and social interactions, we need to learn much more about how amygdala responsiveness may play a role in making a person vulnerable to depression.

Finally, what evidence is available to help us understand the role that the hippocampus, and the other structures that make up the hippocampal formation, might play? Little functional imaging or ERP data yet speak to this question, which represents a clear area of needed research given that we know much about the hippocampal structure's role in long-term memory, attention, and stress responses. However, there is a growing anatomical imaging literature that links hippocampal volume with risk-related factors such as childhood abuse. A smaller hippocampus may impede normal and/or strategic memory functioning. It also may impede the normal feedback mechanisms that happen between critical limbic system costructures such as the amygdala, the hypothalamus, the pituitary, and the adrenal glands, thus having an impact on emotion regulation.

In sum, then, there is evidence that many of the primary brain structures that seem to function abnormally in patients who currently have depression are also different in some way (anatomically or functionally) in individuals who are at greater risk for developing depression. It is not clear if these potential functional or anatomical markers represent more distal or proximal risk factors; the cognitive neuroscience literature has not progressed enough to address this issue. But the research reviewed here does suggest that cognitive neuroscience studies of depression vulnerability may provide powerful and converging empirical tools that could help clarify the diatheses of depression.

7

Cognitive and Cognitive Neuroscience Vulnerability to Depression

Having reviewed cognitive and cognitive neuroscience vulnerability research, we turn now to an integration of these approaches. Despite the cognitive nature of both domains of theory and research, these areas do not always naturally fit together. We start with a discussion of the points of departure for this research and then talk about points of overlap and convergences between the two areas.

POINTS OF DEPARTURE

When comparing two theoretically and empirically distinct domains of research, it is not surprising that the research in these areas are not perfectly overlapping, even when they are trying to understand the same kinds of human experiences. As discussed in the second half of this chapter, there is a good deal of convergence between these literatures. Also for many of the points of departure discussed here, the divergences are positive and productive in that they reflect the fact that each research domain tends to tackle the kinds of problems or questions that are best suited to the empirical tools that each brings to the table. Alternatively, a point of departure can also reflect a need for better "cross-pollination" when an important question is a point of focus in one research domain, but not the other. Thus, one goal of this chapter is to serve this role and try to point out where a concept from one domain might be imported into the other area of research with good effect.

Some of the differences between the cognitive and cognitive neuro-science literatures on vulnerability result from the fact that the cognitive literature has simply had longer to develop. At discussed at length earlier, the diathesis–stress model, hopelessness model, and other cognitive theories of depression are, by psychology standards, quite old. Thus, given the developmental differences between these two literatures, it is arguably very important for researchers from each domain to be fully aware of the progress in the other domain. This cross-disciplinary awareness would serve cognitive neuroscientists well because they would not need to retread ground that had already been well explored. Additionally, cognitive research can look to cognitive neuroscience to help understand some of the possible neural underpinnings of the cognitive and emotional constructs they explore.

As the newer field, cognitive neuroscience approaches to depression can seem less developed. For example, it is a common critique of cognitive neuroscience that the field can be either too methods-driven or too focused on complex correlational data, and thus can be post-hoc in the utilization of theory. An illustrative example of this is the commonly discussed relationship between depression and certain neurotransmitter systems, particularly the catecholamines and tryptamines such as serotonin, first proposed by researchers like Schildkraut (1965).

According to a "monoamine hypothesis of depression," depression arises when low serotonin levels promote low levels of norepinephrine or dopamine. A large portion of the supporting data for this theory comes from the observation that antidepressants that enhance the levels of either norepinephrine or dopamine can impact and reduce the features of depression, leading to the concept that depression is the result of an "imbalance in brain chemicals." However, many would argue that this drug efficacy data does not provide a good bases for developing a neurophysiological theory of depression. As argued by Lacasse and Leo (2005), "this ex juvantibus line of reasoning [i.e., reasoning "backward" to make assumptions about disease causation based on the response of the disease to a treatment] is logically problematic—the fact that aspirin cures headaches does not prove that headaches are due to low levels of aspirin in the brain." There are other problems with inconsistencies in the treatment efficacy data, but even without these problems one must address the question of "What does it mean that a drug like an SSRI causes a reduction in depression symptoms in some patients?" It turns out that this is a very complex question to try to answer. Does this mean that this question should be abandoned? Clearly not, but it will likely take a lot more time and work to develop a theoretically mature explanation for this observed relationship.

One reason that we argue that this kind of underdeveloped theory is, nevertheless, extremely useful is that it has already shown itself to be both empirically and theoretically generative. In part because researchers knew that SSRIs and other related drugs reduced the binding of serotonin to neurotransports, these researchers looked to the gene that encodes this serotonin transporter (found on Chromosome 17) as a possible site for understanding individual differences in serotonin transporter function that might be related to disorders like depression. To date, there have been hundreds of studies of mutations associated with this gene, including the length variations in the *5-HTTLPR* region discussed in some length in Chapters 6 and 8.

A discussion of genetics research leads us to another observation about the differences between the cognitive and the cognitive neuroscience vulnerability literatures, in particular, a difference in the time points that tend to be the focus of each research domain. In examining the research reviewed in Chapters 5 and 6, there seems to be some degree to which the cognitive neuroscientists are more able to focus on a point earlier in human development. Cognitive–clinical research has yet to devise ways to examine potential vulnerability in very young children.

This difference in the temporal aspects of focus are likely in part a reflection of the necessary differences in the methods used by the two domains. Some cognitive neuroscience tools are clearly sensitive to more transient and/or phasic physiological mechanisms that are likely relevant for the study of proximal risk factors. But as discussed in Chapter 6, this kind of research is only now becoming more common. More persistent physiological characteristics that might provide evidence of distal risk factors are more developed research areas (such as the genetics work or the anatomical imaging work assessing the hippocampal or prefrontal cortex systems). Likewise, the cognitive methods discussed include retrospective or recollective techniques that allow for the measurement of distal factors such as parental bonding and childhood abuse. However, it may be the case that current cognitive experience impacts these recollective data to a degree. Thus, without true longitudinal data, it is hard to know the impact that current influences such as cognitive bias or demand characteristics have on measured retrospective data. In short, cognitive distortions might bias a research participant's recollection of her mother's parenting style but they can not impact the current size of the participant's hippocampus. We see this point of departure between the literatures of focus arguing for two things. First, more interdisciplinary research allowing researchers to capitalize on the strengths of both domain's tools and methods would be useful. Second, as discussed in Chapter 4, there needs to be more true longitudinal risk research done using both approaches.

CONVERGENCE IN COGNITIVE–CLINICAL SCIENCE AND COGNITIVE NEUROSCIENCE APPROACHES TO VULNERABILITY

The theoretical foundation of cognitive vulnerability work reflects the convergence of a number of conceptual lines of thought. Obviously Beck's (1967) early theoretical ideas form a core of this foundation, but ideas developed by Ellis (1962) around the same time contribute to this foundation as well. This theoretical framework was also partly built on ideas from learned helplessness and hopelessness as well as by concepts from attachment theory and parental bonding descriptions. Also contributing are broader ideas about the kinds of early experiences that can create or ignite the negative cognition that is at the center of cognitive vulnerability concepts. The theoretical influences and traditions of cognitive–clinical science theories, and the vulnerability predictions that stem from them, are thus varied and intertwined.

Likewise, cognitive–clinical work and cognitive neuroscience share some, but not all, conceptual ancestors. As we noted, cognitive–clinical work, from which much of the cognitive vulnerability literature stems, had its earliest origins in the applied work of Beck and Ellis. Beck noted ideas, however, that were borrowed from cognitive psychology, in particular the concept of schemas. Yet these ideas did not take full advantage of developments in cognitive psychology. Hence the early cognitive–clinical theorizing developed largely in parallel with work in experimental cognitive psychology, and overlapped little. After all, the motive of clinicians was first and foremost to develop effective treatments; articulation and refinement of nascent cognitive theoretical ideas could wait. But the wait was not long. Once the cognitive therapy of depression (Beck, Rush, Shaw, & Emery, 1979) became firmly established, and the cognitive ideas that were attached to this theory seemed to make sense, attempts were made to articulate and refine its cognitive concepts in a fashion that drew from the theories and the methods of experimental cognitive psychology (Ingram, 1986). Contemporary cognitive depression theories are thus the beneficiaries of experimental cognitive work even if this work was not directly linked to the origins of these theories.

Cognitive neuroscience can also be seen as a direct beneficiary of experimental cognitive psychology. That is, a case can be made that experimental cognitive psychology led to cognitive science, which then led to cognitive neuroscience (although along the way of course there were other developments and contributions from other perspectives). Flash forward to today and once again we see some parallel development in the approaches to cognitive depression vulnerability from clinical psychology and from cognitive neuroscience. Fortunately, however, this time the parallel development has not proceded without at least some substantial areas of overlap. This is important in that in areas where there are similarities, cognitive vulnerability work and cognitive neuroscience vulnerability work considered together can compose a more complete and comprehensive picture of depression risk. To be sure, there are differences, but the similarities are meaningful and informative. These similarities can be seen in several domains. One is in the use of diathesis–stress ideas.

Diathesis-Stress Perspectives

Cognitive–clinical science and cognitive neuroscience both make use of diathesis–stress perspectives to inform empirical research. In cognitive vulnerability work this perspective is long established. The first significant research conducted within this framework appeared in 1988 in a study by Miranda and Persons, who found that formerly depressed individuals, after experiencing a mood induction, endorsed greater levels of dysfunctional attitudes than did formerly depressed individuals who did not experience the induction. The mood induction, however, made no difference for never depressed people. The expanding diathesis–stress cognitive vulnerability literature was subsequently reviewed in some detail in 1994 by Segal and Ingram, with a 2005 updated review by Scher et al.

Diathesis–stress research in the cognitive neuroscience literature on depression vulnerability is not as ubiquitous as in the cognitive vulnerability literature, but it is still easy to identify. To cite but one example, Perez-Edgar et al. (2006) failed to find effects for selective attention in the risk group (children of parents with childhood onset) until a negative affective experience (the prospect of giving a speech) was introduced.

As such, this negative experience may be associated with a deficit in selective attention in at-risk children, and may require that more cognitive resources are needed to effectively perform tasks. Such conclusions would not have been possible without a study making use of diathesis–stress ideas.

The adoption of diathesis–stress ideas in both cognitive–clinical science and cognitive neuroscience vulnerability suggests at least two important points. First, from a methodological viewpoint, it seems clear that many important variables, be they defined in cognitive terms or in neuroscience terms, need to be activated before they can be assessed and before diathesis–stress-based theories can be tested. Research has revealed some variables that do not require prior activations (e.g., Hedlund & Rude, 1995), but given that the predominant theories of depression are rooted in diathesis–stress ideas, modeling this relationship in the lab is, and will continue to be, important for most research.

The second point is that the cognitive–clinical and the cognitive neuroscience data together strongly support those theoretical ideas embedded in depression theories, which suggest that emergent depressotypic cognition is a function of stress. Perhaps more importantly, this largely appears to be the case irrespective of the level of cognitive analyses, whether it is reflected in the endorsement of dysfunctional attitudes or seen in the asymmetric activation of the prefrontal cortex. The precise nature of the diathesis–stress link is not clear (i.e., how much vulnerability, how much stress), but at the aggregate level the combination is clearly important. Moreover, as some research has shown, the negative cognition that does emerge is in at least some cases associated with subsequent episodes of depression (Segal et al., 1999, 2006).

Cognitive Similarities between At-Risk and Depressed Individuals

Whether the cognition assessed stems from cognitive–clinical science perspectives or from cognitive neuroscience perspectives, at-risk and currently depressed individuals look similar, provided of course that depressotypic cognition has been appropriately activated. To illustrate the importance of this idea, it may be helpful to revisit elements of a debate that took place in the clinical literature during the last century (which is to say somewhat longer than 10 years ago). Following a number of studies that found evidence of negative cognition in depressed individuals, which sought to draw conclusions about vulnerability (e.g., Ingram

& Smith, 1984), critics responded that this negative cognition might be a consequence of the depression, and thus have not causal relevance (Barnett & Gotlib, 1988). Or that this negative cognition might arise concomitantly with depression, and have no causal relevance. Worse yet for these early cognitive depression studies, research came forth showing that this negative cognition could not be detected in remitted or recovered depressed individuals (Segal & Ingram, 1994).

As we have noted in Chapter 4, none of this research was particularly relevant for understanding depressotypic thinking because these studies did not model the actual complexity of depression theories. Once investigators retuned to these theoretical roots, the "rebirth" of the diathesis-stress perspective put these studies into perspective and showed that, for the vast majority of cognitive variables, activation was needed. Once this activation was included, negative cognition reappeared in nondepressed but vulnerable people. Moreover, as the research we have reviewed has shown, under these conditions, nondepressed but vulnerable people cognitively resemble currently depressed people. To be sure, most research does not include a currently depressed comparison group, but for those studies that do, this cognitive resemblance is similar whether assessed from a clinical perspective or from a neuroscience viewpoint.

Similarities in Cognitive Variables

Although cognitive neuroscience does not have ways to define and measure some constructs (e.g., dysfunctional attitudes, automatic thoughts, irrational beliefs, attributions), nevertheless, there is considerable overlap in the nature of cognitive variables and in their operationalization in research in both areas. More specifically, a good deal of cognitive vulnerability research has relied on the kinds of constructs that are widely understood to reflect basic cognition, and that are articulated conceptually and methodologically by experimental cognitive psychology. We refer in particular to constructs such as memory and attention. Examples across the cognitive and neuroscience spectrum can be seen in efforts to understand the link between selective attention and parental bonding (Ingram & Ritter, 2000) and in the work of Perez-Edgar et al. (2006) who examined selective attention to help understand cognitive resources and task performance in the children of depressed parents. This burgeoning domain of cross-disciplinary research must grow, thus allowing for the study of complex cognitive constructs like attitudes and attributions using the empirically exciting tools of cognitive neuroscience.

Operational Definitions of Vulnerability

Vulnerability can be operationally defined in any number of ways, but not all operational definitions are created equally. That is, some definitions are much more appropriate than others. We discussed this point in some detail in Chapter 2, but this idea warrants some reiteration. For example, it is not appropriate to study risk in already depressed individuals, unless of course the study of risk is aimed at what perpetuates the depressed state. Baring this goal, it is not possible to differentiate between risk factors and those that are consequences or concomitants of the disorder. Operational definitions of vulnerability thus matter.

Fortunately, another area of similarity between cognitive–clinical science and cognitive neuroscience can be seen in operational definitions of vulnerability. Both approaches make use of empirically identified variables. A prime example seen across both approaches is the remission or recovery from depression, reflecting the observation that people who have experienced an episode of depression are at heightened risk for experiencing another episode. Likewise, being the child of a depressed parent is another empirically observable marker that has found its ways into both cognitive–clinical science and cognitive neuroscience approaches. This overlap, to date, has been somewhat intentional and somewhat by chance. As we move forward in the planning of new research, this overlap needs to continue so that comparisons across research domains are possible.

Distal and Proximal Focus

Although framed differently, both approaches investigate distal and proximal vulnerability to depression. In the clinical area, these approaches are reasonably well validated, with origins probably being traced to an explicit discussion of these ideas in the depression arena by Abramson, Alloy, and Metalsky in 1988. These concepts were later elaborated on by Ingram et al. (1998). It is thus not surprising that the terminology in the clinical area makes explicit use of the distal and proximal concepts.

This terminology is not as explicit in cognitive neuroscience research. Nonetheless, examination of cognitive neuroscience studies of vulnerability reveals that some of this research is informative about distal factors and other aspects much more so than for proximal factors. This is the case if we think of research considering genetic measures of potential vulnerability and research done with children that investigates distal factors, or those factors, as we have defined them, that reflect the origins of risk rather than the more immediate precursors of a depressive episode. Indeed, even though these distinctions are not typically used in neuroscience research, some of these studies have investigated even more distal factors than clinical research. Consider, for example, the research by Dawson et al. (1999) and Jones, Field, Davaslos, and Pickens (1997) who examined left-frontal activity in the infants of depressed mothers. To the extent that individual differences in left-frontal hypoactivity exist and predispose children to later depression, or that possible individual differences in the tendency to situationally decrease left-frontal activity are related to depression, this research has the potential to inform us about the neurological origins of adult depression. Clinically motivated research can examine the interactions and draw inferences about how these interactions might create risk, but cannot study possible cognitive vulnerability mechanisms in children this young; it is hard to ask someone to endorse dysfunctional attitudes when they do not yet have attitudes or language. The broader point here is that both clinical science and cognitive neuroscience work focus on proximal and distal vulnerability, and by more explicitly thinking about vulnerability from this proximal versus distal perspective, both cognitive science and cognitive neuroscience researchers will likely have an easier time finding convergence. They will also benefit individually from the greater theoretically specificity that this approach to risk can provide.

SUMMARY

Despite their unavoidable differences, with very little effort cognitive–clinical science and cognitive neuroscience can be thought of as highly compatible and complementary. As we have noted, these approaches investigate very similar phenomena in their focus on cognition, emotion, and depression. Although clinical psychology approached these areas as a means to understand depression, and the cognitive neuroscience interest in emotion led to an interest in depression, both perspectives arrived in the same place.

Cognitive neuroscience can provide some ideas about the areas that are active when certain psychological process occur (e.g., the amygdala is activated during rumination; Siegle et al., 2004). Yet, while cognitive neuroscience can provide important clues as to the neural functioning that is associated with psychological constructs, a one-to-one mapping of the brain functioning underlying a given psychological variable (e.g., dysfunctional beliefs) is unlikely to ever be possible. Nevertheless, taken together, these viewpoints help to provide a more complete picture of the processes involved in vulnerability, and the translation of vulnerability into depression. Indeed, compared to a decade ago, we have considerable knowledge of the psychological variables, and the neural patterns, of vulnerability. Moreover, we can see possible similarities in how these variables operate; for example, there appear to be parallels in at least some of the processes that bring about depression, such as the possible simultaneous deactivation of the left prefrontal cortex and the activation of the depressive self-schema. The brain "location" of such a schema will never be "found," but the combination of cognitive–clinical science and cognitive neuroscience theory and research provide a way that we can understand the same phenomena from different levels of analysis. Certainly, this has enhanced knowledge of depression, depression vulnerability, and, as we will see in Chapters 8 and 9, the treatment and prevention of this disorder. We think it is safe to conclude that depression and depression vulnerability researchers from both traditions look forward to research that continues to bring these levels of analyses together in a manner that will create additional knowledge of depression.

8

Depression Vulnerability and Clinical Therapeutics

If any conclusion is warranted at this point in the book, it is that vulnerability to unipolar mood disorder is multidetermined and set in motion by variables operating across the continuum from neuron to environment. This scope of coverage is helpful as we shift the focus to address the clinical translation of cognitive science and neuroscience accounts of vulnerability and their implications for clinical care. For many patients, their experience with depression and the mental health system in which they receive treatment is defined by the acute episode. Whether treatment is effective, needs to be augmented, or has done its work are questions that usually frame discussions between patient and health care provider. However, a central message in this book is that vulnerable persons require ongoing intervention, a fact that is only now being recognized within the clinical mainstream. In this chapter we review how the data from vulnerability research has highlighted a number of important patient factors that may contribute to effective depression prevention.

One of the benefits provided by empirical studies of vulnerability is that the experimental manipulation of variables of interest can clarify the mechanisms through which depression occurs, is maintained, or returns. As important as this is, the potential for this information to be applied to improve how depression is actually treated or prevented makes it much more valuable. This is because the specificity of the components that comprise treatments for depression, whether pharmacological or psychological, is low. For example, cognitive therapy or interpersonal therapy combine multiple relational, behavioral, and cognitive interventions in the total treatment package, while antidepressant pharmacotherapy targets multiple brain regions in addition to a putative depression circuit (Hollon et al., 2006). The possibility that interventions informed by more precise models of cognitive and neural vulnerabilities to depression could lead to improved patient outcomes has long been one of the field's translational aspirations.

The empirical study of depression treatment and prevention began in the late 1970s and early 1980s and coincided with positive clinical outcomes being reported in randomized trials comparing psychological treatments for depression such as cognitive behavior therapy (CBT; Beck et al., 1979), behavior therapy (Lewinsohn & Hoberman, 1982), and interpersonal therapy (Klerman, Weissman, Rounsaville, & Chevron, 1984) against antidepressant pharmacotherapy (Elkin et al., 1989). These treatments emphasized teaching patients how to deal with stress in their lives, evaluate the accuracy of their interpretations, and learn communication skills and interpersonal problem solving. Using a deductive process of reasoning, the variables suggested as relevant to reducing acute episodes of depression were also thought to play a role in its onset and prevention. Developing prevention treatments that targeted these factors, in either the never depressed, high-risk groups, or vulnerable patients before symptoms emerged, was a logical starting point. In fact, since prevention strategies have routinely been developed by drawing on findings from the depression vulnerability literature, we will now focus on therapeutic applications aimed in part at addressing basic depression vulnerability mechanisms.

PREVENTION OF DEPRESSION
IN SELECTIVE AND TARGETED POPULATIONS

The Institute of Medicine has proposed a tripartite classification of prevention interventions (Mrazek & Hagerty, 1994). According to this system, prevention interventions could be *universal*—delivered to all members of a population and intended to prevent depression onset; *selective*—delivered to subgroups at risk for depression; or *targeted*—delivered to persons demonstrating mild elevations in depression, but falling short of syndromal status. To date, most of the prevention studies in the area of depression have been conducted with indicated populations. As Garber (2008) notes, the findings from these studies have produced small-to-moderate effect sizes, whereas the findings from universal interventions have not shown consistent benefit.

Since the onset for depression can occur during the teen years, and in light of the strong association between negative thinking styles, female gender, and poor coping and episode onset, it should come as no surprise that many depression prevention programs have targeted children and adolescents (Gladstone & Kaslow, 1995; Young & Mufson, 2003). Clarke and colleagues (Clarke et al., 1995, 2001) tested the Coping with Stress Course, a 15-session group intervention emphasizing cognitive restructuring and problem-solving skills, in a randomized trial with ninth- and tenth-grade students who had elevated depressive symptoms. Results indicated a significant reduction in depression scores posttreatment and lower incidence rates of affective disorders up to a year later. In a similar vein, the Penn Resiliency Program (PRP) and it variants (Penn Optimism Program, Penn Prevention Program) have been studied in both younger fifth- and sixth-grade students (e.g., Gillham, Reivich, Jaycox, & Seligman, 1995) and older populations (college students; Seligman, Schulman, DeRubeis, & Hollon, 1999). Of note is the fact that participants were selected not only based on levels of depression but also if they exhibited elevated cognitive risk markers such as a pessimistic explanatory style or dysfunctional attitudes. The findings from this work have reported small-to-moderate effect sizes on depression scores pre- to posttreatment, but benefits tend not to persist over time. Interestingly, changes in cognitive risk markers are also reported, but the extent to which these reductions mediate change in depression is not firmly established. For example, Seligman, Schulman, and Tyron (2007) found that their CBT-based prevention program reduced levels of depression in university freshmen at posttreatment but were no longer evident at follow-up. Participants did, however, report increased optimistic explanatory styles at both these time points.

One consequence of these findings has been a reexamination of the assumptions behind the construction of their prevention programs, namely, their heavy reliance on CBT and behavioral components. One direction that has been advocated is the inclusion of parents in the intervention (Stark, Yancy, Simpson, & Molnar, 2007). Data from Beardslee and colleagues (Beardslee, Gladstone, Wright, & Cooper, 2003; Beardslee et al., 1997) indicated that adhering to a family-based assessment, children of parents with a depressive disorder improved their global functioning and had lower incidence of depression following a clinician-led treatment group compared to a lecture-only group. In a similar vein,

Gillham and colleagues (2006) decided to add a parental component to PRP in an effort to augment outcomes. They reported that a separate six-session intervention for parents led to greater reductions in their children's depressive symptoms over 12 months, compared to controls. Yet these programs remain the exception. Those that exist featuring separate child and parent components are designed to treat acute depression and anxiety states rather than primarily to prevent them (Barmish & Kendall, 2005; Stark et al., 2007).

Another approach to preventing depression is informed by the recognition that since pathways to illness may be multidetermined, patients may benefit from a variety of skills that enable effective prevention—a multicomponent approach. This was borne out in a four-group study conducted by Stice and colleagues (Stice, Burton, Bearman, & Rohde, 2006) who compared four sessions of CBT to a supportive-expressive program of equal length, bibilotherapy, and journaling. They reported reduced depression levels in adolescent participants from pre- to posttreatment in all conditions. Bibliotherapy was the only condition to maintain its gains at a 6-month follow-up. Although the treatment durations in this study were shorter compared to those in other prevention programs (e.g., PRP), the findings suggest that perhaps the normalization of symptoms, destigmatization, and education about depression afforded by each of the interventions had therapeutic value.

The most comprehensive study in this area, and a counterpoint to the arguments for multimodal interventions, was a multisite randomized trial by Garber and colleagues (2009) comparing CBT to usual care in adolescents (ages 13–17) from families in which at least one parent was depressed. The intervention was an 8-week, 90-minute prevention group with six booster sessions and the primary dependent measure was the rate of a probable or definite depressive episode as diagnosed by clinical interviewers. Findings indicated that the hazard of developing depression was lower for adolescents in the CBT prevention program than for those receiving usual care. Of note, whether the participant's parent was depressed at baseline was a significant moderator of the CBT prevention group's efficacy. The CBT prevention program was more effective in preventing onset of depression than usual care for teens whose parents were not depressed at baseline. However, for adolescents with a currently depressed parent, prevention effects between the CBT prevention program and usual care did not differ. The fact that the CBT prevention program had a significant prevention effect through the 9-month follow-up period suggests that its components deserve further study. It also raises interesting questions about how well we understand the process through which these prevention effects were achieved. For example, which of the elements conveyed in each of the CBT group sessions was the most impactful, what concrete skills did participants take away from the course, and was the frequency of practice of prevention skills greater in teens that did not develop depression over the follow-up?

In a related vein, data on depression prevention with an adult focus comes from studies of the "Coping with Depression" (CWD) course, a CBT-based psychoeducational intervention that has been adopted in a number of countries. A recent meta-analysis (Cuijpers, Muñoz, Clarke, & Lewinsohn, 2009) identified six studies in which CWD was employed in preventing new cases of major depression. Its usage was associated with a 38% reduction in the risk of suffering a depressive episode. Since there are likely a number of changes that individuals taking this course make in their lives, we are once again faced with the question of which particular features of CWD were associated with the greatest reduction in depression risk.

Perhaps the most recent development on the prevention front is the use of the Internet to deliver brief psychoeducation and CBT programs for at-risk and mildly depressed persons. In these cases, the prevention link is through the risk of new onsets or the prospect of relapse for someone who was depressed but is currently in remission. One example of Internet-based prevention is Beyond Blue (*www.beyondblue.org.au*), an educational website that offers self-assessment, educational, and self-help resources as they pertain to different affective disorders.

With respect to treatment, three Internet-based CBT websites have received considerable empirical scrutiny. These include (1) Beating the Blues (*www.beatingtheblues.co.uk*), featuring eight 1-hour-long, weekly interactive computer sessions that provide information about depression and CBT strategies to users (Proudfoot et al., 2004); (2) MoodGYM (*moodgym.anu.edu.au*), consisting of five core CBT themes for working with depressive thoughts and feelings that are presented on a weekly basis with an opportunity for revision/summary in the sixth week (Christensen, Griffiths, & Jorm, 2004); and (3) Overcoming Depression on the Internet (ODIN), emphasizing cognitive-restructuring and evidence-gathering techniques delivered in the form of self-guided tutorials (Clarke et al., 2002, 2005). Controlled studies of these interventions compared to either treatment as usual or a depression information website have demonstrated significant effects of the web-based intervention. Specifically, results suggest a modest but reliable improvement in depression scores from pre- to posttreatment on the order of 5 to 6 points on the Center for Epidemiologic Studies Depression Scale (Christensen et al., 2004; Clarke et al., 2005) or 12 points on the Beck Depression Inventory (Proudfoot et al., 2004). Moreover, pre- to posttreatment gains were maintained at 6 and 12 months.

Proudfoot et al. (2004) reported that following completion of Beating the Blues pre–post changes on BDI and Beck Anxiety Inventory (BAI) were maintained over a 6-month interval. Most recently, Mackinnon, Griffiths, and Christensen (2008) found that reduction in depression scores following participation in either MoodGYM or BluePages (another depression information website; *bluepages.anu.edu.au*) were retained 1 year beyond termination and were greater than those for a control condition in which patients were asked questions about their lifestyle. In reviewing this area, Kaltenhaler, Parry, Beverly, and Ferriter (2008) indicated that patients were significantly more satisfied with the Internet CBT programs compared to usual treatment and drop-out rates were generally low, indicating that patients found this format acceptable. Finally, Kessler et al. (2009) reported that patients receiving online CBT and usual care (ten 55-minute sessions during which patients and therapists communicated through online texting) had lower depression scores at 8-month follow-up than a comparison group receiving only usual care from a general practitioner. Taken together, these findings suggest an important role for individually tailored, web-based prevention treatment. Because they can be accessed remotely and have a measurable impact on reducing the intensity of depressive symptoms in at-risk or mildly depressed persons, they may extend the reach of more traditional prevention programs that are hospital-based and largely offered in urban settings.

PREVENTION INFORMED BY NEUROSCIENCE APPROACHES TO DEPRESSION RISK

Although differing in emphasis, a common element shared by the various studies is their reliance on an implicit or explicit formulation of depression risk that is fairly global in nature. Whether mild depressive symptoms, explanatory style, parental depression, dysfunctional attitudes, female gender, stigmatization, lack of knowledge about the condition, or low social support are targeted for intervention, the causal pathway from the point at which these variables are modified to a change in the psychological constructs underlying depression is less well elaborated. A similar argument, but one moving in the opposite direction, can be made about neuroscience findings: at present, they are not sufficiently precise to enable fruitful clinical translation. What is needed is a model of depression risk capable of handling traffic traveling in both directions, from clinical outcomes to neural findings. At present, no such definitive model exits, but there are a number of important findings that can be linked together to outline what this framework would look like and how it might be tested. One key organizing vulnerability construct in such a model is emotion regulation.

According to Werner and Gross (2010), emotion regulation encompasses five types of strategies for regulating an emotional experience at different points in time. *Antecedent-focused emotion regulation* refers to strategies that occur before the experience of emotion (e.g., choosing whether or not to enter a potentially emotion-triggering setting or attending to certain features of a situation over others), whereas *response-focused strategies* describe attempts to influence emotion response tendencies once they have occurred (e.g., constricting facial muscles to prevent oneself from crying). Evidence of impaired emotion regulation in the affective disorders has been extensively documented for the acute phase of illness, and considerable data point to difficulties that persist once depression has remitted (Christensen, Carney, & Segal, 2006; Davidson, Pizzagalli, & Nitschke, 2002). What is the nature of these impairments(s) and how might they be relevant to reducing the risk of depression?

Of note is the finding that initial reactions to negative affect can determine the intensity of subsequent distress, and that there are important differences between the individual regulatory strategies employed (Gross, 2002). In the case of *reappraisal*, in which a negative feeling is recast more optimistically or viewed from a third-person perspective, data suggest that this response can effectively reduce the intensity of fear and anxiety (Ochsner et al., 2004). Yet other regulatory reactions to emotion may be maladaptive, such as *rumination or self-focused attention* in which the cognitive elaboration of negative affect ironically perpetuates the very mood it is intended to reduce (Nolen-Hoeksema, 2000; Watkins et al., 2008). Implementing emotion *regulation strategies that limit the amplification of negative affect* could bolster an individual's ability to cope with depression-inducing events or stressors (Goldin, McRae, Ramel, & Gross, 2008). However, as indicated in a number of the previous chapters, the accessibility of these strategies for at-risk individuals may be lower than for people who have never experienced depression. Interestingly, recent investigations of emotion regulation arrive at a similar conclusion when considering differences in brain function in these populations. Furthermore, the brain structures that have been implicated in this emotion regulation research are the same structures that were discussed in Chapter 6, thus connecting well with the existing anatomical work on depression vulnerability.

Specifically, neuroimaging investigations of emotion regulation have identified a constellation of prefrontal regions associated with active reappraisal of the emotional salience of events (Ochsner & Gross, 2008). Bremner et al. (1997) used short-term depletion of plasma tryptophan to induce a transient clinical relapse in recovered depressed patients and reported a decrease in activity in dorsolateral prefrontal cortex, thalamus, and orbitofrontal cortex in patients who experienced a depletion-inducted relapse but not in those who were below the clinical symptom threshold. Liotti, Mayberg, McGinnis, Brannanm, and Jerabek (2002), however, pointed out that tryptophan depletion is a reliable induction only for a select group of patients, those being treated with an SSRI. They chose instead to employ a cognitive induction method and compared formerly depressed patients, acutely depressed patients, and never depressed volunteers. While induced sadness was associated with decreased activity in medial orbitofrontal cortex for both depressed groups, a reduction in activity in pregenual anterior cingulate was found only in the formerly depressed group.

Of note, these findings were replicated by Gemar et al. (2007) in unmedicated, remitted depressed patients. Other studies have reported that never depressed controls do not show changes during sad mood in these regions using a variety of induction paradigms (Liotti et al., 2002; Mayberg et al., 1999). One hypothesis worth considering is that the presence of these disrupted neural circuits, especially in at-risk populations, may thwart enactment of adaptive emotion regulation strategies.

A candidate mechanism through which sadness-linked changes in the configurations of prefrontal engagement may signal compromised cognitive control over emotion is attentional deployment. Beevers and colleagues (Beevers, Ellis, Wells, & McGeary, 2010; Beevers, Wells, Ellis, & McGeary, 2009; Beevers, Wells, & McGeary, 2009) have conducted a number of innovative studies examining this possibility by using both cognitive tasks and genetic screening to identify at-risk depressed samples, by again examining the serotonin transporter gene promoter region (5-HTTLPR) polymorphism. Recall that this is the same genetic polymorphism that was discussed in Chapter 6 and which has been tied to functional neuroanatomical abnormalities in amygdalar function. In order to understand some of the cognitive implications of this potential genetic marker, Beevers et al. (2010) used a spatial cuing task featuring emotional stimuli to study the relationship between the 5-HTLPPR polymorphism and biased attentional processing in nondepressed adults. They discovered that short 5-HTTLPR allele carriers found it more difficult to disengage their attention from sad and happy stimuli compared with long allele carriers. The fact that this linkage can be found in a nondepressed sample supports the view that susceptibility to depressive reactions in the presence of life stress may involve deficits in attentional deployment when processing emotional stimuli.

Beevers, Wells, Ellis, et al. (2009), further characterized the nature of altered affective processing associated with the 5-HTTLPR polymorphism by looking at other behavioral results of this genetic effect. The investigators employed eye-tracking methodology to examine how individuals genotyped for 5-HTTLPR allocated their attention when simultaneously presented with an array of positive and negative emotional scenes. Their findings indicate that short 5-HTTLPR allele carriers showed a bias toward positive images, whereas long 5-HTTLPR allele carriers were more balanced in their viewing of stimuli with either valence. Homozygotes viewed the stimuli in a more evenhanded fashion. One provocative suggestion is that short allele carriers may be regulating greater reactivity to negative stimuli by intentionally deploying their attention toward positive stimuli. As long as there are attentional resources available to enable this type of shift, the strategy may be adaptive. However, if these resources are reduced by other attentional demands, such as those imposed by dysphoric moods or negative thinking or rumination, vulnerability to depression may increase.

Lastly, Beevers, Wells, and McGeary (2009) unpacked this genetic effect by studying its association with cognitive reactivity following mood challenge. Using a between-groups design, 53 nondepressed participants were genotyped for the 5-HTTLPR gene and assigned to view a sad ($n = 30$) or neutral ($n = 23$) film. Their results indicated that carriers of the short allele increased their endorsement of depressive thinking styles following a sad mood induction compared to carriers of the long 5-HTTLPR allele. The authors suggest that the genetic contribution via 5-HTTLPR allele status to depression vulnerability may be through automatic activation of negative thinking in response to dysphoria-producing events. A similar argument was made by Jacobs et al. (2006) in a 15-month prospective study of 374 young adult female twins. They found that the association between life stress and depression onset was greatest in participants with two short alleles compared to females with one or none. They also found that the effect was moderated by the level of neuroticism, such that it was exhibited most strongly in women who were high on this personality factor. These data speak less to the statistical relationship between the occurrence of a stressor and onset of depression, but more to how an individual's responses to stress and processing of emotional information eventuates in depression. Thus, these data have a strong theoretical link to the alterations in HPA axis function (Jabbi et al., 2007) discussed in Chapter 6. If emotional processing is altered by both the presence of the short 5-HTTLPR allele(s) and level of neuroticism (Keightley et al., 2003), then perhaps interventions designed to enhance mood-linked emotional processing can impact this linkage to the level of depression risk.

In addition to holding a view of vulnerability as the product of poorly modulated reactivity to stressful or dysphoric stimuli, some investigators have conceptualized risk as due to enduring deficits in the processing and consolidation of reward and positive emotion. The basis for this work is the observation that one of the cardinal features of depression is anhedonia, the inability to derive pleasure from activities that were previously enjoyable, and often one of the clinical symptoms that takes longest to return with remission. In fact, a dominant feature of psychosocial treatment for depression is scheduling activities that are intended to restore hedonic capacity.

These deficits have been borne out in studies of depressed patients' neural responses to positive stimuli or reward such as monetary incentives. Epstein et al. (2006) found that, compared to controls, unmedicated depressed patients showed lower bilateral activation in the ventral striatum when positive words were presented. This pattern of activation was also associated with lower ratings of interest or pleasure in the performance of daily activities. Similarly, Heller et al. (2009) reported that differences in frontostriatial regions were associated with depressed patients being less able to sustain positive emotions, compared to controls, while viewing pleasant images.

What is of particular interest is the use of these paradigms with patients in recovery. McCabe et al. (2009), using both the sight and taste of chocolate as a positive stimulus, found that formerly depressed patients showed decreased activations in the ventral striatum compared to healthy controls and that these differences were not a function of the initial ratings of how pleasant, intense, or how much they wanted chocolate. Gotlib et al. (2010) studied 10- to 14-year-old girls who had never been depressed but either had a mother with recurrent depression or no family history. They found that the offspring of depressed mothers showed lower levels of activation in the putamen and left insula but higher activation in the right insula during the anticipation of reward than those in the low-risk group. When negative outcomes were studied, high-risk participants exhibited greater activation in the dorsal anterior cingulate gyrus compared to offspring of never depressed mothers. While further studies are needed to establish the prognostic significance of these results, they may be suggestive of differences in the neural processing of reward and punishment in younger adults at elevated depression risk.

Possible Links between Response to Acute-Phase Depression Treatments and Vulnerability

Although neuroscience studies of mood disorders have led to the identification of possible brain circuits implicated in depression and anxiety, the neural effects of treatments that target these disorders are less well understood (Kessler & Mayberg, 2007). In the depression literature, for example, pharmacological treatments have received the greatest scrutiny, with interest in psychotherapy for depression becoming a focus only more recently. It is possible that knowledge gleaned from a greater understanding of neural pathways associated with effective acute-phase treatment of depression may inform related investigations of relapse or recurrence vulnerability, but that would depend on knowing whether the mechanisms underlying depressive relapse/recurrence differ from those responsible for its reoccurrence in recovered patients. At this point in time, prospective studies of neural markers predictive of depression onset and recurrence are lacking.

The work of Siegle and colleagues is relevant in this context, as it has examined differences in emotion regulation among treated depressed patients, using a measure of the degree of persistence of an emotional stimulus beyond the point of its termination. Clinically, this could be thought of as an analogue to rumination, the tendency to engage in ongoing processing of an emotional event even in the absence of a discrete trigger. Empirically, self-reported rumination has been found to predict depression onset and intensity (Nolen-Hoeksema, 2000). Siegle,

Steinhauer, Thase, Stenger, and Carter (2002) used a cognitive task in which depressed patients received quick presentations of positive, neutral, and negative words (150 msecs) and found evidence of continued processing of negative word content up to 30 seconds after the word had been removed from the screen. Neuroimaging, using fMRI, revealed increased activation in the amygdala in response to this negative information, compared to controls, and decreased reactivity in the subgenual cingulate cortex (Brodmann's area 25; Siegle, Carter, & Thase, 2006). This finding is consistent with what is known about the reciprocal connectivity between these neural regions (as discussed in Chapter 6). The prefrontal cortex has an inhibitory effect on limbic regions such as the amygdala and so decreased activation in dorsolateral prefrontal cortical structures such as the cingulate cortex might lead to sustained amygdala firing and increased emotional reactivity.

Furthermore, reduced reactivity in the subgenual cingulate cortex at pretreatment was specific to patients who received and benefited from CBT for depression. Since a primary goal of CBT is to help patients reduce automatic emotional responding with controlled processing, patients who benefit from this approach may develop increased inhibitory executive control that serves to interrupt more automatic limbic-based responses. When examined closely, many of the functions of the prefrontal cortex that are impaired in depression, such as attentional capacity and cognitive reappraisal, are the targets of therapy intervention in CBT (Goldapple et al., 2004). Strengthening these processes through cognitive assignments and rehearsal may lead to decreased limbic, especially amygdala, activity.

These findings have a number of interesting clinical implications for treatment selection and vulnerability treatment in patients still showing neural reactivity (DeRubeis, Siegle, & Hollon, 2008). First, probing the brain mechanisms that are engaged by psychological (CBT) and biological (antidepressant medication) interventions could lead to treatment algorithms that predict treatment response for individual patients, and differentiate who may be at heightened risk, in spite of apparent remission. Extrapolating from the data presented by Siegle et al., perhaps CBT may be best suited to those patients who demonstrate labile emotional expression or reactivity but who may not be able to engage neural structures to help them temper the intensity of these affects. For those not showing sustained amygdala reactivity, antidepressant medication might be a better first-line treatment. Along the same lines, the presence of sustained amygdale activation to negative words in patients who are judged to be symptom-free might represent an indicator of risk or the need for additional treatment.

Decentering, Metacognition, and the Regulation of Depressive Affect

Mood-linked changes in cognitive processing offer one explanation for why at-risk individuals, whether identified via genotyping, level of cognitive reactivity, depression history, family history, or other markers, become overwhelmed by negative emotion during moments of challenge. Evidence also suggests that compromised prefrontal control over emotion regions may be one reason for the maintenance of habitual or default emotion regulation strategies intended to suppress or avoid dysphoria, but that may unwittingly keep it in place. If we take these findings as a starting point, then perhaps teaching patients to tolerate negative affect without automatically generating elaborative processing routines that characterize this affect as dangerous or emblematic of personal failing might be effective in reducing this reactivity.

Research on ways to reduce automatic response tendencies indicates that shifting attention into a more intentional mode and developing decentering or metacognitive skills may enable greater tolerance and approach of negative affect from a wider attentional frame (Teasdale & Barnard, 1993; Teasdale et al., 2002). Supportive evidence comes from studies in which increased metacognitive awareness of emotions was associated with reduced endorsement of dysfunctional cognitions following sadness challenge (Fresco, Segal, Buis, & Kennedy, 2007), reduced cognitive processing of negative material in present moment awareness (Frewen, Evans, Maraj, Dozois, & Partridge, 2008), and an increased willingness to tolerate negative affect (Arch & Craske, 2006).

Decentering

Decentering has been described as the capacity to take a present-focused, nonjudgmental stance in regards to thoughts and feelings and accepting them. Individual accounts of a decentered relationship to thinking emphasize that one is able to watch thoughts as objects or events in the mind, without being drawn into agreeing with or disputing their content. Thoughts are merely acknowledged as being present in the mind and one can observe them (Safran & Segal, 1990). The construct of decentering, while found in diverse accounts of psychotherapy process (Greenberg,

Ford, Alden, & Johnson, 1993; Horowitz, 1988) has also been featured in conceptualizations of cognitive treatment, suggesting that decentering may reduce levels of depressive rumination by teaching patients more adaptive ways of relating to their thinking. Beck et al. (1979) described it as an important ingredient of change in cognitive therapy and Ingram and Hollon (1986) posited that decentering was not only important in helping to reduce current depression symptoms, but that "the long term effectiveness of cognitive therapy may lie in teaching patients to initiate this process in the face of future stress" (p. 272).

Initial efforts to empirically evaluate the relationship of decentering to depression arose through the study of metacognitive awareness, a construct related to decentering. *Metacognitive awareness* refers to "the process of experiencing negative thoughts and feelings within a decentered perspective" (Teasdale et al., 2002, p. 276). In one of the first reports, Teasdale, Segal, and Williams (1995) assessed 158 patients using the Measure of Awareness and Coping in Autobiographical Memory (MACAM), a semistructured clinical interview, as part of a larger clinical trial. During the acute phase of this study patients received antidepressant pharmacotherapy and those who achieved partial remission of major depressive disorder were randomized to either continue on their medication or take medication together with cognitive therapy for 20 weeks. Results indicated that lower levels of baseline metacognitive awareness predicted earlier relapse across both treatment groups. There was also a larger increase in metacognitive awareness in the cognitive therapy group as compared to the medication-alone group.

Fresco and colleagues' (2007) study of decentering adopted a different tack. They employed a psychometric analysis of the Experiences Questionnaire (EQ), a rationally derived, self-report measure designed by Teasdale to measure both decentering and rumination, not just in affective disorder, but as a more general construct. Using exploratory and confirmatory factor analysis techniques in two consecutive large samples of college students, an 11-item decentering factor emerged. This factor structure was again confirmed in a sample of remitted depressed patients. Findings from this latter sample revealed that healthy controls endorsed higher levels of decentering as compared to recovered patients and that decentering was negatively correlated with levels of both clinician-assessed and self-report symptoms of depression.

An important next step was taken by Fresco et al. (2007) who examined whether treatment response to either CBT or antidepressant medication was associated with gains in decentering and whether such gains moderated the relationship between mood-linked cognitive reactivity and episode return. They reported that increases in decentering, as measured by EQ scores, were found for patients treated to remission with CBT but not for antidepressant medication responders. In addition, higher decentering at the point of remission reduced the association between cognitive reactivity to relapse, such that high decentering and low cognitive reactivity were associated with the lowest rates of relapse over an 18-month prospective follow-up.

Taken collectively, the data from studies in which decentering was assessed directly indicate that patients who are able to develop the capacity to observe their own thoughts and not be drawn into an automatic engagement with their content are better protected against future depression. The challenge for any prevention model is to specify precisely how these skills can be taught. At present, they are understood as consequences of patients achieving a robust response to CBT and possibly other empirically validated treatments for depression. The most reliable way of helping patients to develop decentering skills seems to be through patients receiving one of these treatments. Greater specificity is lacking because decentering is acquired through the larger set of cognitive and behavioral procedures that, if enacted, promote treatment response. Is there a way in which decentering skills could be taught directly (see Figure 8.1)?

Metacognitive Awareness and Mindfulness Meditation

Increases in decentering and metacognitive awareness have been reliably linked to the practice of mindfulness meditation, which is now taught through a number of clinical protocols for the treatment of depression, anxiety, and chronic pain disorders (Kabat-Zinn, 1990; Segal et al., 2002). In fact, the act of simply watching one's experience rather than attempting to alter or control it is central to training in this modality (Brown & Ryan, 2006; Creswell, Way, Eisenberger, & Lieberman, 2007). Of note is the fact that mindfulness as an emotion-regulation strategy differs somewhat from more standard accounts of emotion regulation in the empirical literature that emphasize suppression and reappraisal. *Suppression* attempts to limit the representation of emotion itself (Kim & Hamann, 2007), while *reappraisal* seeks to change the context through which an emotion-inducing stimulus is viewed, thereby altering the subsequent emotional response (Ochsner, Bunge, Gross, & Gabrieli, 2002). Unlike these strategies, however, mindfulness does not

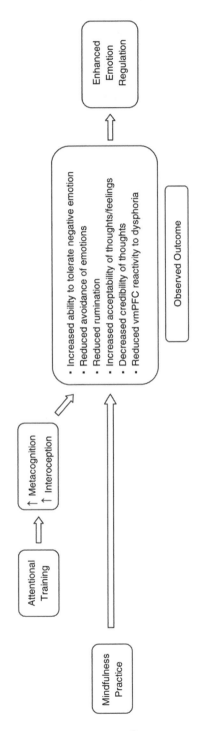

FIGURE 8.1. Mindfulness path to emotion regulation. Adapted from Corcoran, Farb, Anderson, and Segal (2010). Copyright 2010 by The Guilford Press. Adapted by permission.

aim for a desired, nonaversive goal state, but rather attempts to create psychological distance between the emotion and the individual, thereby limiting its behavioral consequences (Kabat-Zinn, Lipworth, & Burney, 1985). Establishing psychological distance from aversive emotions may be part of the reappraisal process (Ochsner & Gross, 2008), but the critical difference is that mindfulness treats the labeling or monitoring of experience as an end unto itself rather than a means by which to then control the emotion (Corcoran, Farb, Anderson, & Segal, 2010).

A core feature of mindfulness practice is the repetitive and deliberate training of attention. This is especially relevant to prevention, as numerous studies have documented differences between individuals at high and low risk for depression in terms of their ability to shift attention toward positive or away from negative emotion stimulus arrays. As described by Lutz, Slagter, Dunne, and Davidson (2008), mindfulness actually encompasses competence in two types of attention foci, labeled "concentrative" and "open." Unlike traditional reappraisal methods, mindfulness training teaches patients to develop moment-to-moment awareness of available stimuli, decoupling the sensory and affective/evaluative aspects of emotion. Through repeated observation of affective states as "objects" of attention (Creswell et al., 2007), patients learn that emotions have their own somatic signatures, whose fluctuations in intensity and duration provide a continuous cue for refocusing attention (Brefczynski-Lewis, Lutz, & Schaefer, 2007), especially when allocation of scarce mental resources to ruminative processing has been the default (Slagter et al., 2007). Indeed, research on practitioners with even brief training in mindfulness has reported evidence for improved attentional control and reduced distractibility (Chambers, Lo, & Allen, 2008; Jha, Krompinger, & Baime, 2007).

Examining the relationship between mindfulness and emotion regulation more directly, Frewen et al. (2008), using a correlational approach, found that individuals high in dispositional mindfulness reported that it was easier for them to disengage from negative thoughts. These associations were replicated in a second study with mildly distressed students who attended an 8-week course in mindfulness training. Participants who evidenced increases in their levels of mindfulness reported decreases in both the frequency and the tendency to ruminate on negative thoughts.

Developing greater metacognitive awareness should result in a shift toward strategies used for dealing with negative internal experiences that reflect a greater openness to, and acceptance of, thoughts and feelings. Indeed, there is evidence that mindfulness training is associated with decreases in maladaptive emotion-regulation strategies such as rumination and avoidance. Ramel, Goldin, Carmona, and McQuaid (2004) found that participants in an 8-week mindfulness training course had lower rumination scores and that these reductions were related to the amount of time participants spent practicing mindfulness. In a laboratory study, mindfulness-based strategies were shown to be more effective in reducing dysphoric mood than strategies involving either rumination or distraction (Broderick, 2005), and decreases in rumination were found to mediate the relationship between mindfulness training and decreased dysphoria (McKim, 2008).

In addition to evidence concerning reducing responses that are positively associated with depression, there is also evidence that mindfulness training may increase behaviors that have a negative relationship with depression, such as a greater ability to tolerate negative emotions and reduced emotional reactivity. Arch and Craske (2006) examined the effects of a 15-minute focused breathing induction on emotional intensity and the participant's willingness to tolerate emotion during a slide-viewing task. Recruitment into the study required that individuals have no prior meditation history and participants were trained to focus their attention on their breathing. Compared to participants in a worry induction and a focused attention condition, participants who followed mindfulness instructions were more willing to remain in contact with highly aversive slides, and they reported less emotional volatility and negative reactivity across the task. Similarly, in a correlational study, Ortner, Kilner, and Zelazo (2007) found that individuals with greater meditation experience reported lower levels of emotional reactivity in response to negative picture slides. In a second study, individuals who completed a mindfulness training program showed increases in mindfulness over the course of treatment, and at posttreatment were found to demonstrate lower emotional reactivity than individuals who had participated in a relaxation course, or those in a wait list condition. These results suggest that another benefit of mindfulness training is that it promotes the ability to disengage from emotionally provocative material, freeing individuals to refocus their attention on other aspects of experience.

From a neuroscience perspective, the distinction between the mindful and the reappraisal approaches to emotion regulation may be better understood with reference to research on pain, where known neural systems underlie the affective and sensory components of pain appraisal (e.g., Singer et al., 2004). While the somatosensory cortices, thalamus, and the posterior insula provide discriminative information about nociceptive stimulus sensation, cortical midline structures such as the anterior cingulate support affective appraisals related to perceived unpleasantness (Craig, 2002). Applying this model, reappraisal processes focus on changing the judgments and evaluation of emotional experience, whereas mindfulness practice focuses attention on emotions as transient sensory responses. Following mindfulness meditation, negative emotions may be experienced more as fluctuations in body state sensations and less as affectively laden mental states reflecting that they are good or bad. Repeated training in adopting this perspective may reduce chronic reactivity by shifting attention away from subjective appraisals of affect toward the incorporation of more sensory-based representations of emotions (Corcoran et al., 2010).

One of the recurring themes in this volume has been characterizing the automatic reactivity, whether behavioral, cognitive, or neural, that at-risk individuals display in the face of mild provocation. Prevention efforts are often designed to counteract this default type of processing. However, it can be difficult for patients to access the cognitive resources necessary to support more adaptive responses without specific training because the default automatic processing has already utilized them. Slagter et al. (2007) examined training effects on the allocation of attention resources in a study employing "attentional-blink," a phenomenon wherein two attentional targets (T1 and T2) presented close in time to each other in a ongoing stream of other targets often leads to the second target not being seen. One explanation for attention-blink is that the two targets are competing for limited attentional resources. Using EEG Slagter and colleagues report a smaller attentional-blink and reduced brain resource allocation to the first target in participants who completed a 3-month program of intensive training in meditation. These are among the first data to suggest that the practice of meditation allows participants some measure of control in how limited cognitive resources such as attention are allocated.

Since attentional deployment is also a hallmark of effective emotion regulation, Lutz et al.'s (2009) study of sustaining attention over longer intervals is particularly relevant. They utilized a dichotic listening task and event-related potentials in nonclinical participants undergoing a 3-month meditation program to examine the impact of this training on the attentional system. Similar to Slagter et al.'s (2007) results, Lutz and colleagues found that the practice of meditation reduced variability in both the attentional processing of auditory tones and reaction times—high variability denotes attentional impairment. The authors concluded that appreciable gains in concentration and sustaining attention can be achieved through meditation.

Clinical accounts describing the benefits of mindfulness practice for regulating negative emotions have stressed that it is not just the effortful switching of attention away from automatic processing routines that is important, but that the lack of judgment of experience is also critical (Kabat-Zinn, 1990; Siegel, 2007; Williams et al., 2007). This type of judgmental stance can often appear in remitted depressed patients as perfectionism or marked self-criticism (Dunkley, Sanislow, Grilo, & McGlashan, 2009; Hawley, Ho, Zuroff, & Blatt, 2006). There are now a handful of studies examining how meditation, particularly practices that support the development of self-compassion in response to criticism, may be useful in regulating these punitive tendencies. Lutz et al. (2008) used affective probes while both experts and novices practiced compassion meditation. They report that the presentation of emotional sounds, such as another's distress, evoked greater pupil dilation and activation of insula and regions of the cingulate cortex, compared to neutral sounds. Between-group differences indicated that experts showed a greater detection and cognitive response to emotional sounds than novices, suggesting that this sensitivity can be acquired through training.

An interesting picture of the neural regions supporting metacognitive and ruminative processing emerges from Farb et al. (2007) who used fMRI to study participants completing an 8-week mindfulness class and novices on a wait list for the same class. In order to investigate mindfulness-linked differences in the capacity for self-reflection, participants were trained in viewing self-descriptive adjectives, while in the scanner, under two cognitive foci, a "narrative" focus, allowing free engagement in self-referential thought, and an "experiential" focus, emphasizing a decentered perspective on the same material. During the narrative focus individuals exhibited distinct engagement of cortical midline structures, including the pregenual dorsomedial prefrontal and posterior cingulate cortices, regions associated with affective appraisals of an event as good or bad for the self (e.g., Northoff & Bermpohl, 2004; Ochsner et al., 2004). By contrast, mindfulness practitioners engaging in an experiential focus exhibited a pronounced shift away from midline cortical activation toward a right-lateralized network comprised of the ventral and dorsolateral prefrontal cortex, as well as sensory representations in the insula and secondary somatosensory cortices. These regions may support more detached, objective interoceptive and somatic awareness

(Craig, 2002) that through repeated observation allow emotions to be viewed as "objects" of attention (Creswell et al., 2007).

Farb, Anderson, and Segal (2010) extended their findings by examining the neural regions supporting emotion regulation during dysphoric mood challenge. Sadness provocation in a mixed sample of depressed, anxious, and chronic pain patients, who were either novices or mindfulness practitioners, correlated with activation along the posterior and anterior regions of the cortical midline, as well as left hemisphere language and conceptual processing centers. These cortical areas are characteristic of cognitive elaboration, increased self-focus, and ruminative problem solving. Sadness provocation was also correlated with widespread deactivations in posterior parietal attentional regions, somatosensory cortex, right insula and right ventral and dorsolateral prefrontal regions, as well as the subgenual anterior cingulate (ACC). In the context of the earlier Farb study, these findings are consistent with the notion of a cognitively evaluative neural network responding to emotion challenge, accompanied by the simultaneous suppression of a viscerosomatic-centered experiential network.

Examining the effects of mindfulness training, the authors found that in the face of equal levels of dysphoric mood, mindfulness practitioners showed less neural reactivity to sadness provocation compared to novices. This effect was observed through both reduced activation of posterior midline and left-lateralized cortical structures, as well as through reduced deactivation of right viscerosomatic networks such as the insula, subgenual ACC, and prefrontal cortex. In particular, mindfulness practitioners displayed reduced activity in the posterior midline regions associated with autobiographical memory retrieval and self-referential processing, and in classical language areas (left posterior superior temporal gyrus and left frontal operculum). The recovery in the mindfulness group of novice-observed deactivations in the insula and subgenual ACC has also been observed in the recovery of patients with mood disorders (Goldapple et al., 2004). The authors conclude that the combination of reduced posterior midline and language network recruitment, as well as recovered viscerosomatic activity, following mindfulness training suggests reduced self-evaluation and increased nonevaluative viscerosomatic representation of sensation and emotion. With respect to depression prevention, the body of literature reviewed, including this last study, suggests that training in mindfulness may serve to restore the neural balance between evaluative and interoceptive activity during sadness, approximating that of the nondysphoric state.

IMPLICATIONS FOR THE DESIGN OF DEPRESSION PREVENTION INTERVENTIONS

Although insufficient by itself as a prevention strategy, training patients in mindfulness skills may be invaluable as a part of procedures to "nip in the bud" incipient relapse (Teasdale et al., 1995). Such procedures share with existing CBT techniques the aim of helping patients "decenter" from negative automatic thoughts and feelings and can be combined with training in utilization of basic CBT techniques to produce a novel treatment specifically designed for the prevention of future relapse in patients who have already recovered from depression as a result of either pharmacotherapy or cognitive therapy and other empirically supported psychotherapies. One important difference between this approach and currently existing models of CBT delivery posttreatment (either in booster sessions or maintenance mode) should be highlighted. In the latter model, patients are encouraged to prepare for future stressful events by rehearsing and augmenting their repertoire of coping behaviors. Examples of this would include performing a situational risk analysis, identifying cognitive triggers, and saving records from therapy that can be pulled out and reviewed in response to a stressor. This approach is largely episodic and relies on warning signs of the episode's appearance for its enactment.

An alternative approach emphasizes acquiring control over a cognitive process that is used on a daily basis (attention) and as such is not tied to the occurrence of potentially distal adversity. Training in mindfulness can be mastered during periods of euthymia so that the patient can be more adept at using it when difficult situations occur. This format is consistent with the needs of a maintenance treatment since the work the patient is expected to do is continuous with recovery and can begin following the completion of acute treatment. Finally, because training in mindfulness is nonpharmacological and addresses mood outcomes in a broader context of well-being, it may appeal to remitted depressed patients who may be wary of continued intervention.

SUMMARY

Although knowledge generation has always been central to the scientific enterprise, when it comes to domains of study in which empirical findings bear on health outcomes, their clinical translation is a vital part of this process. In this chapter, we reviewed the evidence for mechanisms of depression vulnerability found in comparative depression treatment studies, with an eye toward factors that were associated with the maintenance of treatment gains. The bulk of studies featured CBT, and from this work the importance of changes in metacognitive processing and the ability to decenter, or adopt an "observer" stance on experiences was noted as being particularly promising. Measures of these constructs have been validated and it was suggested that training in mindfulness meditation may be one avenue for teaching these skills to patients directly.

9

Prevention Efforts
Designed to Address Factors
Underlying Depression Risk

As we have seen in the previous chapter, while knowledge of depression risk factors can certainly inform targets of therapeutic focus, they alone do not comprise a clinical protocol for preventing depression. In this chapter we review recent work that has sought this integration, including describing these treatments and their clinical outcomes. What is especially noteworthy is the importance placed on the linking the presence of depression risk factors to skills for teaching patients how to dismantle the bias they introduce or on finding ways of compensating for it.

As discussed earlier, interventions for preventing depression have been designed on the basis of information from a variety of sources including the efficacy of treatments for acute depression spawning versions of the same treatment delivered during remission (Frank et al., 1990), knowledge of risk factors associated with depressive relapse (Segal et al., 2006), and differences in the incidence of depression between young males and females (Garber et al., 2009). The range of prevention interventions is diverse and features individual, group, or web-based treatment formats for populations that include never depressed, previously depressed but currently remitted, remitted patients with recurrent depression, and patients in partial remission.

In reviewing work in this area, Hollon et al. (2006) suggest that a cross-cutting theme relevant to all prevention treatments is the mechanism through which their outcomes endure. Indeed, Hollon et al. (2006)

differentiate between two kinds of enduring effects. The first type refers to *treatment effects*, factors that address and reduce problems that would have persisted but for structured intervention. Treatment effects of prevention interventions can be assessed by whether the problem they are supposed to target does or does not reoccur or, if it reoccurs, that its frequency and/or intensity is reduced compared to pretreatment. An intervention that is truly *curative* would work by eliminating or reversing the underlying processes that would otherwise lead to the continuation of the disorder. The second type refers to *preventive effects*, an intervention's capacity to reduce future risk for the problem—presumably by undermining the causal processes that could result in the disorder's onset or recurrence. The value of viewing prevention outcomes from this perspective lies in its suggestion that some posttreatment changes may be reflective of symptom reduction, whereas others may bear on reduction of illness and future risk. This classification may be helpful to keep in mind as we consider the state of treatments used to prevent depression and whether their outcomes more closely resemble treatment or preventive effects.

APPROACHES TO DEPRESSION PROPHYLAXIS

In the broadest terms, two strategies to achieve prophylaxis in depression have been dominant: extending the treatment provided during the acute phase beyond the point at which symptoms have improved or employing acute treatments that have effects that endure beyond the point at which treatment is terminated (Segal, Pearson, & Thase, 2003).

Temporal Extension of Acute-Phase Treatment

The value of continuing treatment beyond the disappearance of depressed symptoms was initially signaled by high rates of recurrence following antidepressant medication withdrawal after initial symptom relief (Oltman & Friedman, 1964). This view has gained considerable acceptance, as seen in current practice guidelines that emphasize the need to continue treatment for between 6 months to 1 year beyond the timeframe of full or partial resolution of affective symptoms (American Psychiatric Association, 2000) and up to 3 years for patients who suffer from recurrent depression. The premise behind discriminating acute from maintenance treatment is that the mode of action of antidepressant drugs is symptom-suppressive, and does not target the putative pathophysiology of the episode itself (Hollon et al., 2006). Maintaining patients on antidepressant medication throughout the expected duration for an episode of major depressive disorder ensures that the underlying mechanisms driving the disorder will run their course, while causing a minimum of disruption in the patient's life. Supportive data for this position comes from studies that have compared continuation treatment with either an antidepressant or a placebo, following acute response. In general, 50–70% of the placebo-treated patients developed depressive symptoms meriting a diagnosis of major depressive disorder, compared to only 20–30% of the medication-treated patients (Glen, Johnson, & Shepherd, 1984; Kocsis et al., 2007).

In addition to maintenance antidepressant pharmacotherapy, different forms of psychotherapy have been shown to be of value in preventing depression. The pioneering work of Frank and colleagues (1990) in modifying an empirically validated depression treatment, interpersonal therapy (IPT), to enable monthly rather than weekly sessions, is a good example. They studied 128 patients who, after being treated with the combination of imipramine and IPT, achieved remission and were randomized to one of five prevention conditions: placebo, placebo plus IPT, IPT alone, imipramine alone, and imipramine plus IPT. Patients continuing on imipramine had the longest survival over a 3-year period but there was also a modest prevention effect for IPT. The fact that IPT lengthened the time between episodes, compared to patients not receiving an antidepressant, suggests its utility in that not unsizeable number of patients who whether due to side effects, pregnancy, or motivation cannot continue on long-term antidepressant treatment.

Using a similar strategy, Jarrett and colleagues (2001) reported on a continuation form of cognitive therapy (C-CT) in which the same therapist administering acute-phase CBT provided 10 additional sessions over 8 months. The focus in these sessions was on using emotional distress or symptoms to activate the skills learned during acute-phase CBT to regulate depressive experiences. Over a 2-year follow-up, relapse rates for C-CT were 10% while patients receiving only acute-phase CT relapsed at a rate of 31%.

Enduring Effects of Acute-Phase Treatments

A second strategy for protecting patients against episode return is the use of acute treatments whose effects endure beyond the point of treatment termination. Studies comparing the long-term outcomes of patients who recovered following acute-phase cognitive therapy (CT) with the outcomes of patients who recovered and who were then withdrawn from antidepressant medication have consistently found less relapse or need for further treatment in the CT group (Blackburn, Eunsun, & Bishop, 1986; Evans et al., 1992; Shea et al., 1992; Simons, Murphy, Levine, & Wetzel, 1986). While critiques of this work have questioned the adequacy of antidepressant medication delivery in the earlier studies and possible differential attrition, the general pattern of findings is consistent.

The most comprehensive study to date comparing CT and antidepressants for preventing depression, and one designed to specifically address these methodological shortcomings, was conducted by Hollon et al. (2005). These investigators recruited moderately to severely depressed patients and treated them either with medication or with CT during the acute phase of their depression. Patients who remitted were then randomized to either discontinue their medication and receive a placebo, continue on their medication, or discontinue CT. Hollon et al.'s data show that rates of relapse following continuation pharmacotherapy (42%) and acute-phase CT (31%) did not differ but both were significantly lower than placebo (76%). This lends further support to the idea that acute-phase psychological treatments may have long-lasting effects in reducing depressive relapse risk, presumably through patients acquiring skills, or changes in thinking, that confer some degree of protection against future onsets.

Some Limitations on the Use of Monotherapies for Preventing Depression

All the studies reviewed to this point in the chapter have employed monotherapy, the reliance on a single treatment modality over the course of care, in the service of prevention. While the efficacy data for maintenance pharmacotherapy and psychotherapies is welcome news for both patients and practitioners, this approach does have its drawbacks.

An operative assumption behind the use of maintenance pharmacotherapy is that patients are required to take their medication for extended periods. However, in practice this plan is compromised by rates of patient noncompliance in the 40% range (Basco & Rush, 1995). In one study of 155 depressed outpatients, 28% stopped taking antidepressants during the first month of treatment and 44% had stopped taking their medicine by the third month (Lin et al., 1995), well short of the duration recommended for ensuring sustained improvement. The issue of patient noncompliance is a complex one. While many patients discontinue because of negative experiences with their medication, such as fatigue from side effects, others, ironically, discontinue because of symptom or functional improvement, feeling that treatment is no longer needed (Demyttenaere et al., 2001; ten Doeschatte, Bockting, Koeter, & Schene, 2009). Patients' decisions to initiate and continue with antidepressant medication face two challenges at different time points. Early default may reflect side-effect burden or lack of response whereas later default may be a product of treatment response (Trivedi et al., 2007). At minimum, these data indicate that prevention via compliance with a multiple-year antidepressant medication regimen would lose a significant number of at-risk individuals.

A second alternative, of providing acute-phase, structured psychotherapies, such as CBT and IPT, on a large scale may also prove to be difficult and not feasible (Olfson et al., 2002). Treatment delivery depends on scarce, expensive, professionally trained personnel. It may not be possible to deliver these interventions, in their traditional formats, to make much of an impact on an illness as prevalent as depression. Alterations to their traditional formats, such as the move to computer-aided interactive treatments, in which the level of individual therapist contact is reduced, has been one response to these resource limitations (Osgood-Hynes et al., 1998).

Most importantly, perhaps, is the observation that patients in the acute versus the remission phases of depression have different needs and seek the types of care that best correspond to these challenges (Fava, Tomba, & Grandi, 2007). One fundamental assumption behind relying upon the same treatment both to achieve acute-phase remission and to ensure prophylaxis is that the mechanisms responsible for the return of symptoms during remission are the same as those maintaining the symptoms during the acute episode. In the realm of somatic treatments, this assumption is largely supported by survival rates of 70–80% of patients receiving maintenance pharmacotherapy (Frank et al., 1990; Hochstrasser et al., 2001). For psychological treatments, however, this assumption may be less justified. As we have stressed throughout this volume, a cognitively informed analysis of relapse vulnerability (see also Alloy et al., 2006; Ingram et al., 1998) highlights the difference between the processes involved in relapse, namely, the reactivation of an enduring depressogenic cognitive structure, and those processes that maintain the depressive episode, which are primarily recruited once this structure is activated. This suggests that prophylactic treatments designed with this distinction in mind will differ in emphasis and appearance from those primarily designed to alleviate established depression.

Provision of Prophylactic Treatment to Patients Already in Remission Following Acute Treatment

A more promising approach to prevention than monotherapy is the use of sequenced, phase-specific treatments for depression (Fava, Ruini, & Rafanelli, 2005). This approach has received far less attention than the other two approaches described above. The use of lithium carbonate in conjunction with acute-phase antidepressant treatment is one example of its clinical application. Greil et al. (1996) evaluated the prophylactic efficacy of lithium (LI) and amitriptyline (AMI) in recurrent unipolar depression over a period of 2.5 years. All patients received acute-phase antidepressant medication and were then either continued on AMI or discontinued and started on LI. Greil et al. found that both LI and AMI were equally effective in preventing recurrences and that there were no differences in hospitalization rates between the two groups. In fact, LI tended to outperform AMI in prevention of "subclinical recurrences." A recent Cochrane Database review of lithium's role as a maintenance treatment for mood disorders (Burgess et al., 2001) concluded that lithium prophylaxis was more effective than placebo in preventing relapse in mood disorders overall, and especially in bipolar disorder.

Another strategy sequences pharmacologically induced remission with psychological prophylaxis of relapse/recurrence, thereby taking advantage of the cost-efficiency of antidepressant pharmacotherapy in reducing acute symptomatology while providing a psychological intervention during recovery to reduce the subsequent risk of depressive relapse or recurrence. The data recently generated by studies employing this approach suggest that it has considerable promise in helping patients achieve durable outcomes following recovery from depression.

Blackburn and Moore (1997) studied 75 recurrently depressed patients assigned to one of three groups: acute- and maintenance-phase antidepressant treatment, acute- and maintenance-phase CT, and acute-phase antidepressants followed by maintenance-phase CT. Results indicated that all treatments reduced depression levels in the acute phase and there were no differences in relapse prevention between the groups. This was among the first studies to demonstrate maintenance CT has a similar prophylactic effect to maintenance medication in pharmacologically remitted patients. Similarly, Paykel et al. (1999) reported that for patients who showed only a partial response to pharmacological treatment, adding a 20-week course of CT significantly lowered relapse rates compared to patients who continued to receive standard pharmacotherapy alone. Bockting et al. (2005) developed a group CT approach that could be offered to remitted depressed patients regardless of their medication status. The program comprised eight weekly sessions with a focus on the identification and modification of dysfunctional attitudes and group participants were compared against control patients receiving usual care over a 2-year follow-up. Results indicated no difference between the groups, but a secondary analysis found a benefit for group CT in patients who had experienced five or more depressive episodes.

The work of Fava and colleagues (Fava, Grandi, Zielezny, Rafanelli, & Canastrari, 1996; Fava, Rafanelli, Grandi, Conti, & Belluardo, 1998) provides some of the most encouraging preliminary evidence for the efficacy of a sequenced, phase-specific approach to prophylaxis in depression. Using a similar design across two studies, the Fava groups compared outcomes for pharmacologically treated depressed patients who, following remission, were discontinued from medication and received either clinical management or a hybrid form of CT. For remitted patients who exhibited some residual symptoms, relapse rates in the CT group were 35% at 4 years and 50% at 6 years, while those in the clinical management condition relapsed at 70% and 75%, respectively. Group differences at the 4-year follow-up were statistically significant, but were no longer so at 6 years. However, when the total number of depressive episodes over the 6 years was calculated, patients receiving CT had experienced significantly fewer episodes.

Modifying Acute-Phase Psychological Treatment for Prophylactic Intervention during Remission

As has been described, most of the psychotherapies employed as continuation or maintenance treatments for depressive relapse prevention required some modification from their acute-phase versions. In its simplest form, this has resulted in fewer therapy sessions over a fixed time period (Blackburn & Moore, 1997; Frank et al., 1990), which addresses the need to deliver treatment over a longer follow-up period or to provide less intensive treatment to patients no longer in episode. In these studies the prophylactic treatment is essentially the acute-phase treatment administered less frequently. However, as we have previously argued, prophylactic treatments designed for use with remitted patients should differ in emphasis from those primarily designed to alleviate established depression. This principle is already implicit in some of the studies reviewed earlier. For example, in the Jarrett et al. (2001) and the Bockting et al. (2005) studies, the emphasis was on identifying relapse vulnerabilities and generalizing coping strategies acquired during acute CT.

A more extensive modification of an acute-phase treatment is found in the approach taken by Fava (Fava et al., 1996, 1998). The theoretical background for his CT-based prophylactic treatment is derived from care strategies used with patients suffering from chronic, recurrent medical illness, such as cardiovascular disease, asthma, or diabetes. In all these disorders lifestyle changes can have a significant impact on health. Patients in Fava's program are told that depression is the consequence of a maladaptive lifestyle that discounts the powerful effects of stress, interpersonal friction, overwork, and poor sleep habits on precipitating relapse. They are asked to reduce such inappropriate lifestyle behaviors and to replace them with activities that will enhance well-being and personal meaning in their lives. CT techniques for addressing residual symptoms such as anxious or irritable moods are also taught. The addition of lifestyle modification and well-being components to standard CT is intended to increase CT's relevance to patients in recovery and increase compliance among those feeling that their level of functioning precludes the need for preventive care.

Fava's studies are noteworthy as being among the first to apply a theoretical understanding of the nature of relapse mechanisms to the modification of an already effective acute-phase treatment so as to address these mechanisms more directly. Conceptualizing prevention of depressive relapse as analogous to lifestyle management of other chronic medical illnesses provides a useful framework for developing effective prophylactic interventions.

An alternative, and perhaps more direct, approach would be to develop prophylactic interventions that specifically target the cognitive mechanisms that underlie depressive relapse. The past few years have produced a marked increase in our understanding of the nature of cognitive risk for relapse in depression (Alloy & Riskind, 2005; Ingram et al., 1998) and it is possible that treatments informed by this understanding will be more effective in addressing relapse mechanisms. A recently developed prophylactic treatment that uses this strategy involves combining training in mindfulness meditation with the principles of cognitive therapy: mindfulness-based cognitive therapy (MBCT). Before proceeding to describe this intervention, it is instructive to consider some of the neural findings that would support this particular type of integration.

MINDFULNESS TRAINING AND THE NEURAL CORRELATES OF SADNESS REACTIVITY AND RELAPSE

A suggestion made in the previous chapter was that training in mindfulness has the dual effect of reducing activation of evaluative posterior midline and language regions in the brain, while restoring activity in areas subserving viscerosomatic representations of sensation and emotion. This in essence may help restore a neural balance between these regions that approximates the nondysphoric state and makes it easier for patients to enact adaptive coping strategies to deal with real-world challenges. These findings, however, have come from studies that have looked at cross-sectional differences between groups and have not reported on actual relationships to depression outcomes. Two fMRI studies using longitudinal and pre–post designs present data relevant to this initial hypothesis.

Farb, Anderson, and Segal (2010) studied 16 formerly depressed patients who had been successfully treated with an antidepressant and were then followed for 18 months to evaluate their relapse status. Using the same sadness provocation paradigm as Farb, Anderson, Corcoran, et al. (2010), they replicated the finding that transient induced dysphoria activated areas in the medial prefrontal cortex and led to deactivations in more lateral regions including the posterior insula and superior temporal gyrus. This pattern was significantly associated with the number of past depressive episodes and, most importantly, to relapse status. Neural reactivity to sadness in the dorsal and ventromedial prefrontal cortex predicted relapse status, suggesting maladaptive reactivity in this region in response to emotional stressors, whereas neural reactivity to sadness challenge in the right anterior insula/operculum *negatively* predicted relapse, suggesting a protective reactivity in response to emotional stressors.

Using a between-groups pre–post design, Farb, Anderson, Corcoran, et al. (2010) examined changes in attentional capture by mood-congruent and mood-incongruent stimuli, under conditions of sad and neutral mood induction before and after mindfulness or relaxation training. Participants were asked to make judgments about whether a photograph depicted an indoor or an outdoor setting. Each photograph had a transparent human face superimposed on it with each face exhibiting either a neutral or a sad expression. This task has been used to assess the degree of automatic emotional processing imposed by different mood states. In this case the interest lay in measuring the interference associated with a negative face when making an indoor/outdoor image decision during sad mood. Results indicated that reaction times for all participants got quicker when the task was readministered under neutral mood at posttreatment, but that only participants in the mindfulness group responded more quickly at posttreatment when tested under sad mood. Furthermore, these changes in the mindfulness group were associated with increased activation in the right anterior insula, a region that has been implicated in the nonevaluative, interoceptively based representation of emotions. These data are among the first to suggest that training in mindfulness may promote more flexible emotional processing and resilience to emotional challenge distinct from the benefits of nonspecific support or relaxation. Based on these findings, the incorporation of mindfulness training for a more comprehensive treatment package designed to prevent depressive relapse/recurrence would certainly be warranted.

Prevention of Depressive Relapse with MBCT

Broadly conceptualized, mindfulness is a way of paying attention that permits thoughts and feelings to be observed as events in the mind, without overidentifying with them, and without reacting to them in an automatic, habitual manner. This is thought to introduce a "space" between one's perception and response that favors *reflective* versus *reflexive* responses to situational demands (Kabat-Zinn, 1990; Shapiro & Carlson, 2009). An operational definition of mindfulness offered by Bishop et al. (2004) defines a two-component model featuring (1) attentional self-regulation of immediate experience and (2) an orientation of acceptance and curiosity toward mental contents. These two elements have been identified in numerous accounts of the intersections between mindfulness and psychotherapy (Germer, Siegel, & Fulton, 2005; Hayes & Feldman, 2004) and empirical support for these two components has been based on behavioral (Anderson, Lau, Segal, & Bishop, 2007) self-report (Lau et al., 2006), and neuroimaging (Farb et al., 2007) data.

Mindfulness is typically developed through various meditation techniques that originate in Buddhist spiritual practices (Hanh, 1976) but have recently been introduced in a secular format that permits their practice without any religious or spiritual connotation (Brach, 2003). Of note, there has been a surge of interest over the past 10 to 15 years in the clinical use of mindfulness including, in particular, the integration of mindfulness with cognitive-behavioral psychotherapies. Two main approaches have been taken toward training mindfulness in a clinical context, although it is important to add that they are not mutually exclusive. First, mindfulness-informed psychotherapy employs a theoretical framework that reflects insights derived from both Buddhist and Western psychology, as well as the therapist's own personal practice. Mindfulness-informed treatments include Martell, Addis, and Jacobson's (2001) behavioral activation treatment for depression and Hayes, Strosahl, and Wilson's (1999) acceptance and commitment therapy. In the second case, mindfulness-based psychotherapies explicitly educate patients in the practice of mindfulness. These treatments can vary in the relative emphasis of mindfulness training over other therapeutic elements. In dialectical behavior therapy (DBT; Linehan, 1993), a treatment for borderline personality disorder (BPD), some formal meditation practice is incorporated, but it is limited in scope, in part due to minimal low capacity or willingness of this patient group to tolerate their internal experiences for long periods. Mindfulness-based stress reduction (MBSR; Kabat-Zinn, 1990), on the other hand, is an intensive 8-week program of training in mindfulness that is almost entirely based on formal and informal instruction and practice of mindfulness. MBCT (Segal, Williams, & Teasdale, 2002) would be situated somewhere in the middle as it combines training in mindfulness with CT techniques.

Empirical Support for MBCT in Preventing Depressive Relapse

To date, the empirical status of MBCT has been examined in four randomized controlled trials. The first multicenter trial ($n = 145$; Teasdale et al., 2000) was conducted at three sites (Toronto, Canada; Cambridge, England; Bangor, Wales), while the second trial ($n = 75$; Ma & Teasdale, 2004) was a single-site replication (Cambridge, England). In both trials, individuals had to be in remission and off medication for at least 3 months before they were randomized to receive either MBCT or to continue with treatment as usual (TAU). In the MBCT group, individuals participated in eight weekly group sessions plus four follow-up sessions and were then followed for a year. The primary outcome measure was whether and when patients experienced relapse or recurrence defined as meeting DSM-III-R criteria for major depressive disorder. In both trials, the samples were stratified according to the number of previous episodes (one or two vs. three or more). The results from the first study revealed a significantly different pattern of results for individuals with two versus three or more episodes. For those individuals with only two previous episodes (23% of the sample), the relapse rates between the MBCT and TAU groups were not statistically different. On the other hand, for the group with three or more episodes (77% of the sample), there was a statistically significant difference in relapse rates between patients receiving MBCT (37%) compared to TAU (66%) over the study period. Similarly, Ma and Teasdale (2004) reported relapse rates for individuals with three or more depressive episodes (73% of the sample) of 36% for MBCT versus 78% for TAU whereas there was no prophylactic advantage of MBCT for individuals with a history of only one or two depressive episodes. Taken together, these two studies show that for patients with recurrent major depression who had experienced three or more previous episodes, MBCT halved rates of relapse/recurrence over the follow-up period.

Two more recent studies provide additional evidence for the efficacy of MBCT. Bondolfi et al. (in press) conducted a French language replication of Ma and Teasdale's (2004) study with 60 unmedicated depressed patients in remission who had experienced at least three past episodes. While no difference in relapse rates between the two groups was reported, over a 14-month prospective follow-up, time to relapse was significantly longer with MBCT + TAU than TAU alone (median 204 and 69 days, respectively). In addition, analyses of homework frequency suggested that MBCT patients, compared to TAU, made active use of skills taught in the program to regulate sad moods. Finally, Kuyken et al. (2008) conducted a parallel two-group randomized controlled trial comparing patients with recurrent depression on maintenance antidepressants with those receiving MBCT. Over a 15-month follow-up, relapse rates were 47% for MBCT and 60% for the antidepressant group, indicating that MBCT afforded protection on par with the current standard of care. Moreover, patients in MBCT had significantly lower residual depressive symptoms and higher quality-of-life ratings over the follow-up than did patients continued on medication. These data suggest that MBCT, with its emphasis on a set of daily therapeutic tasks that emphasize awareness and mood regulation, may be easily integrated into patients' lifestyles over the long term in ways that help to protect against relapse and to support improved quality of life (ten Doesschate, Koeter, Bockting, Schene, & DELTA Study Group, 2010).

While these results support MBCT's efficacy in reducing depressive relapse, the study designs used to date do not permit ruling out confounding explanations for the treatment benefits, such as group support, destigmatization, and/or therapeutic attention. There is indirect support, however, for the finding that the effects of MBCT are consistent with the underlying theoretical rationale. The demonstration that MBCT was more effective than TAU for individuals with a history of three or more episodes is consistent with the view that MBCT helps individuals disrupt autonomous relapse processes that involve the automatic reactivation of depressogenic thinking patterns by dysphoria at times of potential relapse. Convergent with this finding is the finding that MBCT was more effective than TAU for depression onsets where no antecedent major life stressors were reported but that there was no difference between MBCT and TAU for depressive episodes that were preceded by a major life stressor (Ma & Teasdale, 2004).

Commonalities between Prophylaxis Mechanisms in CT and MBCT

At present, CT has the strongest empirical evidence for prevention of relapse/recurrence in patients who were treated for the acute phase of the illness (Hollon et al., 2005). It would seem a logical starting point for the design of any stand-alone prevention treatment to understand how CT might achieve these effects. In Beck et al.'s (1979) original cognitive model, depression vulnerability was related to underlying dysfunctional attitudes that remained unmodified during treatment, carrying the possibility that these dormant beliefs could be retriggered in remission by life stress. From this, it would follow that CT reduces relapse risk by modifying dysfunctional attitudes (Garratt, Ingram, Rand, & Sawalani, 2007). An alternative, but not incompatible, view offered by Ingram and Hollon (1986) proposes that CT has its prophylactic effects by facilitating the individual's ability to "decenter" or "distance" from his or her depressive thoughts such that they are no longer seen as absolutely true. While the concept of "decentering" had been recognized in previous discussions of CT (e.g., Beck et al., 1979), it typically had been viewed as simply a means to the end of changing the content of thinking, for example, from biased to balanced. However, it is possible that the very

CT skills that patients acquire through homework practice mimic learning in mindfulness-based treatments about how to develop a new relationship to negative automatic thoughts.

Let us take a closer look at the modal intervention used in CT, the Daily Thought Record. This seven-column form allows a patient to catch automatic thoughts that arise in the context of an emotional shift and to then consider the evidence for and against their line of thought. Later columns enable these sources of evidence to be synthesized into a more balanced thought and to rerate the intensity of negative emotion (Beck et al., 1979). Successful use of the Thought Record leads to changes in the degree of belief in negative automatic thoughts and is associated with treatment response (Tang, DeRubeis, Hollon, Amsterdam, & Shelton, 2007). Approaching from a slightly different vantage point, it is possible to view the first three columns as training patients in accepting and tolerating negative affect in an effort to approach and become curious about internal experiences—essentially a shift from an automatic mode of responding to one that is more intentional and effortful. Similarly, the columns asking for evidence that supports/does not support the "hot thought" encourage a decentered perspective on thinking itself, as the patient evaluates the thought as an "idea" of what is occurring, rather than the reality of the situation itself. Is it a stretch to say that CT teaches patients a mindful way of relating to thoughts and feelings? Perhaps not.

Of course, to be fair, it is possible that the clinical effects of MBCT derive from the teaching of CT skills to patients in the program. Could it be that once patients are able to practice mindfulness in the context of negative affect, they are better prepared to engage in types of cognitive (re)appraisal efforts that are fostered in CT and that this is what is ultimately protective? This hypothesis is difficult to rule out in the absence of studies comparing these two interventions directly, or without dismantling studies in which only a portion of the core skills are taught, compared to the full-package treatment.

One important difference between MBCT and CT, however, has to do with the phase during which the skills are taught. In CT, patients learn these skills in the presence of low mood and depressive symptoms, whereas a treatment designed for use with remitted patients must be able to do this regardless of mood state and symptom picture because these features may not be pervasive in their lives. This is one of the aims for which MBCT was designed. We now describe how this is achieved.

THE 8-WEEK MCBT PROGRAM

Participants' first exposure to the MBCT program comes during an initial interview and orientation session with the instructor. This is as much of a chance for the rationale behind MBCT to be conveyed as it is for the instructor to let the participant know about the practice demands that come with attending the classes. Patients learn that MBCT integrates aspects of mindfulness-based stress reduction (Kabat-Zinn, 1990) with standard CT techniques and that they will engage in formal mindfulness meditation practices such as the body scan, mindful stretching, and mindfulness of breath/body/sounds/thoughts, as well as informal practices that encourage the application of mindfulness skills in everyday life (e.g., eating a meal mindfully, monitoring physical sensations, thoughts and feeling during pleasant and unpleasant experiences). The CT strategies include psychoeducation about the symptoms that denote depression, the types of automatic thoughts commonly reported by depressed patients, and exercises designed to illustrate the ABC model of thoughts and feelings and how the nature of one's thoughts can change depending on the situation. Patients also learn to nominate activities that provide them with a sense of mastery and/or pleasure as well as create a specific relapse prevention plan. In order to facilitate the practice of these skills between sessions, MBCT introduces patients to the 3-minute breathing space, a miniaturized meditation, to facilitate present-moment awareness during stressful situations (Segal et al., 2002). Finally, participants in the MBCT program are asked to engage in a daily meditation practice and homework exercises directed at integrating these skills into daily life. Viewed in its entirety, the skills taught in MBCT can facilitate awareness of negative thinking patterns with an accepting attitude that enables the individual to respond in a flexible and deliberate way to these thinking patterns at times of potential relapse, a response style that runs counter to the ruminative, judgment-based problem solving identified in previous chapters as increasing depression risk. What follows is a brief description of how these goals are accomplished over the course of the 8-week treatment.

Awareness of Present Experience with Acceptance

The first four MBCT sessions are devoted, in large part, to facilitating nonjudgmental awareness of present experience. This is accomplished via the formal meditation practices, which in generating both pleasant and unpleasant reactions help participants to learn a number of important skills including concentration; awareness of thoughts, feelings, and bodily sensations; and returning to present-moment experience. Many patients see their reactions to things happening around them in terms of an undifferentiated amalgam of positive or negative feedback. In MBCT patients start to develop the ability to deconstruct such experiences into their component elements of physical sensations and the accompanying thoughts and emotions. Awareness of depression-related experience is also emphasized and patients are provided with handouts describing the diagnostic criteria for major depression, as well as the Automatic Thoughts Questionnaire (Hollon & Kendall, 1980) to familiarize them with the types of negative thinking that can occur in depression in order to facilitate their early detection.

Recognizing "Doing and Being" Mode

A core feature of the program involves facilitation of an aware mode of being, characterized by freedom and choice, in contrast to a mode dominated by habitual, overlearned "automatic" patterns of cognitive-affective processing. For patients, this distinction is often illustrated by reference to the common experience, when driving on a familiar route, of suddenly realizing that one has been driving for miles "on automatic pilot," unaware of the road or other vehicles, preoccupied with planning future activities or ruminating on a current concern. By contrast "mindful" driving is associated with being fully present in each moment, consciously aware of sights, sounds, thoughts, and body sensations as they arise. When mindful, the mind responds afresh to the unique pattern of experience in each moment, rather than reacting "mindlessly" to fragments of a total experience with old, relatively stereotyped, habitual patterns of mind. Increased mindfulness allows early detection of relapse-related patterns of negative thinking, feelings, and body sensations, so allowing them to be "nipped in the bud" at a stage when this may be much easier than if such warning signs are not noticed or are ignored. Further, entering a mindful mode of processing at such times allows disengagement from the relatively "automatic" ruminative thought patterns that would otherwise fuel the relapse process. Formulation of specific relapse/recurrence prevention strategies (such as involving family members in an "early warning" system, keeping written suggestions to engage in activities that are helpful in interrupting relapse-engendering processes, or to look out for habitual negative thoughts) are also included in the later stages of the program. Following the initial phase of eight weekly group meetings, follow-up meetings are scheduled at intervals of 1, 2, 3, and 4 months.

Similarities and Differences between CT and MBCT

As the name suggests, MBCT shares similarities with more traditional CT. The most important of these is the focus on relapse prevention, which depends on identifying triggers and potential warning signs of an incipient relapse as well as developing an action plan of how the patient can best take care of him- or herself in this event. Other similarities include a focus on educating patients about the symptoms of depression including the experience of automatic thoughts, monitoring thoughts and feelings in unpleasant situations, and rating activities for the degree of pleasure and mastery they evoke.

However, MBCT significantly differs from CT in a number of important ways. The most important difference is MBCT's emphasis of an acceptance-based approach versus CT's change-based orientation. This distinction is important to consider because it maps onto an earlier point regarding the needs of persons who are depressed differing from those in recovery (Fava et al., 2007). To illustrate the difference between acceptance and a change-based approach, consider the negative thought "I am unlovable." Mindfulness practice invites the person to notice this thought as an event occurring in the mind rather than as a truth that defines the self, but noticing does not involve changing how much one believes it to be true. It can merely be acknowledged as "Oh, there is that thought again" and then returning attention to the task at hand. In contrast, CT involves the evaluation and the possibility of restructuring cognitions and beliefs in the service of acquiring more functional ways of viewing the world. In this case, a person having the same thought might recall important counterexamples of being unlovable and respond "There is not a lot of support for this way of looking at things because my wife told me the other day that she loved me." The point here is that patients who are in the midst of a depression need to learn how to evaluate their thinking styles for evidence because the automatic thoughts are "louder" and persist, even after they are noted and labeled. In remission, however, automatic thoughts are not as "loud," and therefore adopting an approach that emphasizes curiosity and approach may be sufficient to allow the person to disengage from the thought's content or command.

SUMMARY

In this chapter we examined the rationale for, and clinical outcomes from, prevention treatments designed on the basis of teaching patients to address depression risk factors. What is interesting about this work is that the risk factors are not the more common clinical and demographic variables such as treatment adherence or social support, but reflect the acquisition of psychological skills for identifying, reappraising, and regulating mood states. Whether through the deliberate use of thought records in cognitive therapy or the attentional training featured in mindfulness meditation, the empirical data point to significant prevention outcomes when these interventions are offered once acute treatment for depression has ended. Having defined and surveyed the broad scope of research on vulnerability and its clinical application, we now turn to consider the implications of these literatures at the level of the vulnerable person.

10

The Vulnerable Person Revisited

In the Preface to this volume, we described the characteristics of a prototypical vulnerable person. We described her as a woman to denote that gender is a risk factor, but as we discussed in Chapter 2, risk is not the same as vulnerability; risk tells us about probability and vulnerability tells us about process. Possessing a vulnerability factor, of course, means that the person is at risk and thus, as we also noted, vulnerability is most properly seen as a subset of the broader category of risk factors.

But what makes our individual vulnerable? When we ask for her assistance in studies, it may be because she was depressed in the past, and as we know from Chapter 4, this means that she is at risk for being depressed again. Or it may be because she had a depressed mother, which also places her at risk for depression. Of course, having a depressed father may be as problematic as having a depressed mother, and it is even more likely problematic if both parents are depressed, although we cannot say this with certainty because by and large only depressed mothers are studied.

WHAT MAKES A PERSON VULNERABLE?

Because of the assistance of vulnerable people in research efforts, we know there are a number of variables associated with vulnerability, but of course our explorations in this volume have focused on cognitive science and cognitive neuroscience approaches to vulnerability. These approaches are conceptually closely associated in that cognitive neuroscience focuses on the brain structures, connections, and processes associated with cognition, and cognitive–clinical approaches emphasize psychological experiences and processes that can be thought of as part of the "mind." However, even though they are closely linked at a conceptual level, cognitive–clinical work and cognitive neuroscience have largely proceeded in parallel with less contact than is scientifically desirable. Despite these separate histories, these approaches have nevertheless helped us to understand the functions of vulnerability to depression.

Cognition

What does thinking look like in our vulnerable person? Despite some subtle cognitive differences, when our vulnerable person is not depressed her thinking does not look all that different from a person who is not vulnerable. However, cognitive theories suggest, and the data support, the idea that vulnerable individuals possess negatively toned self-schemas that have links to the mechanisms responsible for the activation of sad affect. As the data examined in Chapter 5 show, such schemas are not fully operational during times of stability or emotionally quiescent functioning for vulnerable individuals. Yet these cognitive structures become the first response to negative events. This seems particularly to be the case to the extent that events are appraised as negative, personally meaningful, and (most likely) interpersonal. Thus, despite the largely emotionally benign cognitive functioning that is seen in the vulnerable person in a normative state, negative cognitive structures are activated by various triggering events.

Several broad themes appear to be represented in these activated schemas. As we examined in Chapter 5, these themes involve conceptions of the self that are negative, unfavorable, or derogatory in nature, which reflect core beliefs that are activated when the depressive self-schema is brought online. The pervasiveness of this negative belief system may also help mediate the frequency at which these themes are activated. That is, although we have suggested that these schemas are latent until activated, individuals with particularly extensive and well-connected negative personal belief systems may facilitate the activation of these beliefs to the overt level. For instance, the person who has an extensive self-schema anchored by beliefs of personal inadequacy may be more likely to perceive verification of this inadequacy in interpersonal functioning, whether such verifying data exist or not. If, for example, the person with a well-elaborated sense of inadequacy is on heightened alert for cues of inadequacy in social situations, then such cues may be found and interpersonal difficulties may be generated. Thus, in addition to serving to interpret events in a depressive manner, these structures may also play a role in the creation of activating events.

Cognitive Neuroscience of Vulnerability

Just as various thinking proclivities characterize the vulnerable person, so too do various brain functions. As we reviewed in Chapter 6, cognitive neuroscience approaches have generated a considerable amount of data, and shed a considerable amount of light, on brain function in the depressed state. To the extent that neuroscience researchers have been interested in vulnerability, much of their speculation and theorizing about risk has come from studies of currently depressed patients. As we have seen, however, while studies of depressed individuals might provide important clues, vulnerability cannot be directly studied, because the presence of depression (or significant negative affect), confounds vulnerability work. To establish vulnerability, variables must be present or identifiable before the episode, that is, temporal antecedence must be demonstrated.

There has been some neuroscience research, however, that has directly examined vulnerability, and for that reason we highlight it here. Perhaps the most solid evidence of brain function in our vulnerable person is evidence of cingulate gyrus and left prefrontal cortex hypoactivity. As we have noted, however, a question arises as to whether such hypoactivity is chronic in nature or rather that the vulnerable individual has a propensity for quick hypoactivation in response to stress. The prefrontal cortex, for example, appears to play a key role in regulating other structures that are involved in the neural circuitry of the acutely depressed state. To play a role in vulnerability, then, it may be the case that rather than chronic hypoactivation, prefrontal cortex hypoactivity is a reaction to stress. In some respects this can be seen as analogous to the depressive cognitive schema in vulnerability. It is not the chronic activation of such a schema that makes our person vulnerable but rather the schema's presence and ability to be activated in response to stress. Thus, for the prefrontal cortex, it may not be its hypoactivation so much as its ability to become quickly hypoactive. Ultimately, research will need to examine which of these scenarios is more accurate.

The other brain region that appears clearly implicated by risk research is the limbic system, particularly the amygdala and hippocampus. Evidence for the role of the hippocampus comes primarily from studies examining differences in the size of the hippocampus in vulnerable individuals, with the hippocampus being smaller in our vulnerable person. This is significant because the hippocampus is seen as important for modulating activity in the amygdala, just as the amygdala likely impacts the episodic memory functions carried out by the hippocampus. Moreover, indirect evidence comes from the fact that studies show biased or disrupted memory processes in our vulnerable person, and the hippocampus (along with other medial temporal lobe structures) are critical for mediating episodic long-term memory functions.

With regard to the amygdala, research has examined its function in vulnerable individuals and found shifts in amygdala activation in response to negative affective stimuli. These data thus suggest that activation (or the facilitation of activation) plays a role in what makes the vulnerable person vulnerable. Given the amygdala's role in the experience of emotion, and the fact that ruminative thinking has also been linked to amygdala activation, it is not surprising that research has identified this region as a potentially important contributor to vulnerability. As with hypoactivation of the prefrontal cortex (and possibly because of this hypoactivation), it may be the ease of activation rather than a chronically activated state that characterizes the nondepressed but vulnerable individual.

Thus from the perspective of cognitive neuroscience, the issue for our vulnerable person may be that, when encountering stress, hypoactivation of the left prefrontal cortex and the cingulate gyrus is coupled with too much activation of the amygdala and a failure of the hippocampus to modulate this amygdala activity effectively. As a result, the negative mood that is associated with the stressful event is amplified and the vulnerable person is less able to engage in effortful, prefrontally mediated, compensatory strategies that might help to repair mood. As the negative mood state is further potentiated by these processes, neural regulatory mechanisms become compromised and eventually the neural circuitry of depression becomes fully engaged. Our vulnerable person has now gone from vulnerable to experiencing a major depressive episode.

ORIGINS OF VULNERABILITY

If our picture of vulnerability is accurate, how does this risk arise? Taken chronologically through the person's lifetime, first consider the genetic factors that might help to put our vulnerable person at risk before she is even born. Pre- and postnatal development of the brain involves a complex series of precisely timed stages that are subdivided into the generation, migration, and differentiation of neurons. Components of monoaminergic neurotransmitter systems participate in this brain development, and therefore help set the stage for normal brain function and, likely, for psychopathology. There is an increasing body of evidence indicating that the serotonin transporter regulatory system is critical in the genesis, differentiation, and maturation of networks in the brain that are important for interpersonal interaction, emotional, and stress responses. A range of research has found that carriers of the abnormal *5-HTTLPR* allele may be less efficient in regulating serotonin reuptake at the presynaptic neuron. Given serotonin's role in regulating neural circuits that subsume the processing of emotion information, such differences may explain why abnormal *5-HTTLPR* allele carriers are more likely to respond to life stress with depressive reactions as at least some vulnerable people later develop their prototypical emotional response patterns. It is clearly not the case that all vulnerable individuals are at increased risk because of an abnormal genetic profile, but this potential origin of vulnerability is important for at least some people who will eventually develop depression. Research will be important to determine not only how genetic profiles confer risk, but also how people with such profiles become resilient against depression.

What are the environmental or experiential events that likely impact our vulnerable person after she is born? As we noted in Chapter 5, the data strongly suggest that vulnerability is tied to negative events in childhood. In particular, sexual abuse is an event that is associated with future depressive episodes, yet, as we also noted, not all sexually abused children will eventually become depressed, and not all individuals who experience depression were sexually abused. Thus, sexual abuse is an important variable, but beyond a specific type of stress like sexual abuse, which kinds or categories of stressful events might lead to vulnerability to depression? It seems reasonable to suggest that negative events that occur in abundance, are chronic or very traumatic, occur in the context of multiple and likely interacting domains (e.g., a very dysfunctional family, divorce, high levels of poverty, problematic peer relationships) will impact vulnerability. Not all such events necessarily have depression-vulnerability-producing effects, nor are events such as these the only progenitors of depression-predisposing processes, but they seem like reasonable candidates to profoundly affect the neural connections, learning processes, and what is learned by the developing child in ways that create vulnerability.

Most broadly, a case can be made that when these types of events disrupt attachment and parental bonding they appear to be associated with vulnerability. For instance, at least at the overt level, diminished parental care clearly seems to play a role in the origins of vulnerability. This lack of care can be reflected by emotional neglect in some cases, or in others by chronic or intense criticism or abuse. Indeed, the potential long-term effects of negative events are likely to be particularly virulent when they involve key attachment figures. As a result, the child may not only begin to develop working models that are comprised of cognitive representations of current or future significant others as neglectful or unreliable, but also develops a cognitive structure that represent the self as unworthy of attention and care and as deserving of punishment and poor treatment.

Given the context in which these cognitions arise, negative affect is likely to become entwined with their development. Thus, cognitive self-structures potentially become closely linked to sadness affective structures through this developmental process. Negative affect, therefore, becomes not only intricately connected with unfavorable views of the world and others, but strongly associated with unfavorable conceptions of the self. The soon-to-be vulnerable-to-depression person thus develops a schema of the self as unlikable and unlovable that is strongly tied to the experience of negative affect. When individuals with these cognitive/affective links encounter sadness-producing experiences in the future, they not only experience negative emotions, but, given the close connections, also activate a variety of negative cognitions concerning the self. In sum, negative events, particularly as they are related to attachment figures, can have a profound effect on the child's developing cognitive/affective networks. Not only is the content of the individual's core belief systems negatively toned, but this is consolidated in the formation of increasingly intricate and complex neural associations and connections. Some of these connections may reflect the propensity to hypoactivate prefrontal processes and to activate the limbic system. The processes that are affected by negative events in childhood thus set the stage for the role of negative events in initiating depression in the future. However, as we note in Chapters 8 and 9, given these processes, it is not surprising that many effective methods for treating depression and vulnerable people aim to decouple cognition and negative affect and, in so doing, to reactivate self-regulatory neural circuits.

STRESS (AND EVOLUTION)

Throughout the research we have reviewed, we have emphasized the importance of a diathesis–stress framework. Having just summarized the diathesis part of this equation and its origins, we turn now to the kind of stress that engenders the transition from vulnerability to depression. Most broadly, we suggest that a key kind of stress for the vulnerable person reflects interpersonal loss, that is, the dissolution of an emotionally bonded relationship. Other types of negative events may initiate depression as well, but interpersonal loss is especially problematic situation for a person vulnerable to depression. A probable reason that this is because we are hard-wired by our evolutionary history toward the maintenance of bonds with others, and when these bonds are broken an aversive emotional state is created.

Indeed, it is not an evolutionary accident that interpersonal loss is one of the most powerful precipitants of depression; we are genetically and biologically wired not only to seek out interactions with others in general, but to seek out intimate interactions with at least some people. This idea was first advanced in the context of attachment processes by Bowlby in 1961 in that the capacity to experience sadness has evolutionary survival value; if the loss of a significant interpersonal relationship brings on an aversive state of sadness, this state serves as a motivator to reestablish the relationship where possible, or if not possible, to seek out new relationships. We are thus genetically predisposed to feel an aversive state when losses are suffered, and similarly predisposed to attempt to relieve this aversive state by redeveloping (if possible) preexisting bonds, or if not possible, by developing significant new social bonds.

The establishment of these emotional bonds and significant relationships with others helps to ensure the survival of the species in that not only are individuals who are affectively motivated to create interpersonal bonds more likely to reproduce, but if we examine the protracted helplessness experienced by human infants, those who have the benefit of emotionally bonded parents are more likely to survive and pass on attachment-linked/sadness genes to their offspring. As Bowlby (1988) summarized:

> It is ... more than likely that a human being's powerful propensity to make these deep and long-term relationships is the result of a strong gene-determined bias to do so, a bias that has been selected during the course of evolution. With this frame of reference, a child's strong pro-

pensity to attach himself to his mother and father, or to whomever else may be caring for him, can be understood as having the function of reducing the risk of his coming to harm. For to stay in close proximity to, or in easy communication with, someone likely to protect you is the best of all possible insurance policies. Similarly, a parent's concern to care for his or her child plainly has the function of contributing to the child's survival ... and thereby the [survival of the] individual's own genes. (pp. 81, 165)

The core element of depression, sadness, thus has evolutionary value. If, however, the interpersonally linked sad state is accompanied by the prior development of negative self-schemas, and a propensity to hypoactivate the cingulate gyrus and left prefrontal cortex, and to hyperactivate the limbic system, then the normal negative affect state is set to spiral into a depressive state. Indeed, if loss is interpreted in terms of one's own inadequacy and inferiority, this becomes reminiscent of Freud's differentiation between mourning and melancholia: in mourning the person's response to a loss is "This is terrible," in melancholia the person's response to this loss is "I am terrible." And as proactive behaviors are diminished by hypoactive neural structures while negative affect and rumination is amplified by limbic structures, the normal negative affective state that has evolved for adaptive functioning ("This is terrible") instead becomes maladaptive ("I am terrible"). The vulnerability function of the mechanisms we have outlined therefore lies in the transition from a normal and short-term negative affective state into a prolonged depressive psychopathological state.

FINAL COMMENT

There are many ways to examine the interaction between cognitive and neurocognitive variables and depression. Indeed, numerous books have been published, hundreds of research findings have been reported, and thousands of people have volunteered their time to be studied. As we examine this work in the cognitive and neurocognitive domains, we have attempted to capture some of the essential elements of the interaction between these processes as they apply to vulnerability considerations. To do so, we have examined the nature of depression and have reviewed both research and research methodologies that apply to the study of depression. We have also examined possible origins of vulnerability and have discussed treatment considerations as well. In this chapter we have attempted to summarize this information to develop a concise but accurate picture of how certain forms of cognitive and neurocognitive functioning render some people at risk for depression. As such, our discussion of these topics and ideas reflect our cognitions, and only time and research will tell us whether these cognitions are distorted, or rather reflect some reality about vulnerability to depression.

References

Abela, J. R. Z., & Hankin, B. (2008). Cognitive vulnerability to depression in children and adolescents: A developmental psychopathology perspective. In J. Abela & B. Hankin (Eds.), *Handbook of depression in children and adolescents* (pp. 35–78). New York: Guilford Press.

Abramson, L. Y., & Alloy, L. B. (1990). Search for the "negative cognition" subtype of depression. In D. C. McCann & N. Endler (Eds.), *Depression: New directions in theory, research, and practice* (pp. 77–109). Toronto: Wall & Thompson.

Abramson, L. Y., Alloy, L. B., & Metalsky, G. I. (1988). The cognitive diathesis–stress theories of depression: Toward an adequate evaluation of the theories' validities. In L. B. Alloy (Ed.), *Cognitive processes in depression* (pp. 3–30). New York: Guilford Press.

Abramson, L. Y., Metalsky, G. I., & Alloy, L. B. (1989). Hopelessness depression: A theory-based subtype of depression. *Psychological Review, 96,* 358–372.

Abramson, L. Y., Seligman, M. E. P., & Teasdale, J. (1978). Learned helplessness in humans: Critique and reformulation. *Journal of Abnormal Psychology, 87, 49–74.*

Adolphs, R., Damasio, H., Tranel, D., & Damasio, A. (1996). Cortical systems for the recognition of emotion in facial expressions. *Journal of Neuroscience, 16,* 7678.

Agency for Health Care Policy and Research (*AHCPR*). (1993). Depression in Primary Care: Vol. 1. Detection and Diagnosis. Clinical practice guideline number 5 (DHHS Publication No. *AHCPR* 93–0550). Washington, DC: U.S. Government Printing Office.

Ainsworth, M. D. S. (1989). Attachments beyond infancy. *American Psychologist, 44,* 709–716.

Ainsworth, M. D. S., Blehar, M. C., Waters, E., & Wall, S. (1978). *Patterns of attachment: A psychological study of the strange situation.* Hillsdale, NJ: Erlbaum.

Akiskal, H. S. (1987). Overview of biobehavioral factors in the prevention of mood disorders. In R. F. Muñoz (Ed.), *Depression prevention: Research directions.* Washington, DC: Hemisphere.

Alloy, L., Abramson, L., Safford, S., & Gibb, B. (2006). The Cognitive Vulnerability to Depression (CVD) Project: Current findings and future directions. In L. Alloy & J. Riskind (Eds.), *Cognitive vulnerability to emotional disorders* (pp. 33–61). Mahwah, NJ: Erlbaum.

Alloy, L., Abramson, L., Tashman, N., Berrebbi, D., Hogan, M., Whitehouse, W., et al. (2001). Developmental origins of cognitive vulnerability to depression: Parenting, cognitive, and inferential feedback styles of the parents of individuals at high and low cognitive risk for depression. *Cognitive Therapy and Research, 25,* 397–423.

Alloy, L. B., & Abramson, L. Y. (1979). Judgment of contingency in depressed and nondepressed students: Sadder but wiser? *Journal of Experimental Psychology: General, 108,* 441–485.

Alloy, L. B., & Abramson, L. Y. (1982). Learned helplessness, depression, and the illusion of control. *Journal of Personality and Social Psychology, 42,* 1114–1126.

Alloy, L. B., Abramson, L. Y., Grant, D., & Liu, R. (2009). Vulnerability to unipolar depression: Cognitive-behavioral mechanisms. In K. Salzinger & M. R. Serper (Eds.), *Behavioral mechanisms and psychopathology: Advancing the explanation of its nature, cause, and treatment* (pp. 107–140). Washington, DC: American Psychological Association.

Alloy, L. B., Abramson, L. Y., Whitehouse, W. G., Hogan, M. E., Panzarella, C., & Rose, D. T. (2006). Prospective incidence of first onsets and recurrences of depression in individuals at high and low cognitive risk for depression. *Journal of Abnormal Psychology, 115,* 145–156.

Alloy, L. B., Hartlage, S., & Abramson L. Y. (1988). Testing the cognitive diathesis–stress theories of depression: Issues of research design, conceptualization, and assessment. In L. B. Alloy (Ed.), *Cognitive processes in depression* (pp. 31–73). New York: Guilford Press.

American Psychiatric Association. (2000). *Diagnostic and statistical manual of mental disorders* (4th ed., text rev.). Washington, DC: Author.

Amir, N., McNally, R., Riemann, B., Burns, J., Lorenz, M., & Mullen, J. (1996). Suppression of the emotional Stroop effect by increased anxiety in patients with social phobia. *Behaviour Research and Therapy, 34,* 945–948.

Ancy, J., Gangadhar, B., & Janakiramaiah, N. (1996). "Normal" P300 amplitude predicts rapid response to ECT in melancholia. *Journal of Affective Disorders, 41,* 211–215.

Andersen, S. L., & Teicher, M. H. (2004). Delayed effects of early stress on hippocampal development. *Neuropsychopharmacology, 29,* 1988.

Andersen, S. L., & Teicher, M. H. (2008). Stress, sensitive periods and maturational events in adolescent depression. *Trends in Neurosciences, 31,* 183–191.

Anderson, J. (1985). Ebbinghaus's century. *Journal of Experimental Psychology: Learning, Memory, and Cognition, 11,* 436–438.

Anderson, C. A., & Hammen, C. (1993). Psychosocial outcomes of children of unipolar depressed, bipolar, medically ill, and normal women: A longitudinal study. *Journal of Consulting and Clinical Psychology, 61,* 448–454.

Anderson, N. D., Lau, M. A., Segal, Z. V., & Bishop, S. R. (2007). Mindfulness-based stress reduction and attentional control. *Clinical Psychology and Psychotherapy, 14,* 449–463.

Aneshensel, C. S. (1985). The natural history of depressive symptoms: Implications for psychiatric epidemiology. *Research in Community and Mental Health, 5,* 45–75.

Angold, A., & Costello, E. (1998). Puberty and depression: The roles of age, pubertal status and pubertal timing. *Psychological Medicine, 28,* 51–61.

Arch, J. J., & Craske, M. G. (2006). Mechanisms of mindfulness: Emotion regulation following a focused breathing induction. *Behaviour Research and Therapy, 44,* 1849–1858.

Armitage, R. (1995). The distribution of EEG frequencies in REM and NREM sleep stages in healthy young adults. *Sleep, 18,* 334–341.

Armitage, R., & Hoffmann, R. F. (2001). Sleep EEG, depression and gender. *Sleep Medicine Reviews, 5,* 237–246.

Aserinsk, E. (1968). Length of rapid eye movement (REM) state of human sleep. *Federation Proceedings, 27,* 224.

Aserinsk, E. (1973). Relationship of rapid eye movement density to prior accumulation of sleep and wakefulness. *Psychophysiology, 10,* 545–558.

Avery, D. H., Holtzheimer, P. E., Fawaz, W., Russo, J., Neumaier, J., Dunner, D. L., et al. (2006). A controlled study of repetitive transcranial magnetic stimulation in medication-resistant major depression. *Biological Psychiatry, 59,* 187–194.

Avis, N. (2003). Depression during the memopausal transition. *Psychology of Women Quarterly, 27,* 91–100.

Baker, J. T., Sanders, A. L., Maccotta, L., & Buckner, R. L. (2001). Neural correlates of verbal memory encoding during semantic and structural processing tasks. *Neuroreport, 12,* 1251–1256.

Bandura, A. (1969). *Principles of behavior modification.* Oxford, England: Holt, Rinehart, & Winston.

Banks, S. M., & Kerns, R. D. (1996). Explaining high rates of depression in chronic pain: A diathesis–stress framework. *Psychological Bulletin, 119,* 95–110.

Barber, J. P., & DeRubeis, R. J. (1989). On second thought: Where the action is in cognitive therapy for depression? *Cognitive Therapy and Research, 13,* 441–457.

Barmish, A. J., & Kendall, P. C. (2005). Should parents be co-clients in cognitive-behavioral therapy for anxious youth? *Journal of Clinical Child and Adolescent Psychology, 34,* 569–581.

Barnett, P. A., & Gotlib, I. H. (1988). Psychosocial functioning in depression: Distinguishing among antecedents, concomitants, and consequences. *Psychological Bulletin, 104*, 97–126.

Bartholomew, K., & Horowitz, L. M (1991). Attachment styles among young adults: A test of a four-category model. *Journal of Personality and Social Psychology, 61*, 226–244.

Basco, M. R., & Rush, A. J. (1995). Compliance with pharmacology in mood disorders. *Psychiatric Annals, 25*, 269–275.

Batgos, J., & Leadbeater, B. J. (1995). Parental attachment, peer relations, and dysphoria in adolescence. In S. Goldberg, R. Muir, & J. Kerr (Eds.), *Attachment theory: Social, developmental, and clinical perspectives*. Hillsdale, NJ: Analytic Press.

Beardslee, W. R., Bemporad, J., Keller, M. B., & Klerman, G. L. (1983). Children of parents with major affective disorder: A review. *American Journal of Psychiatry, 140*, 825–832.

Beardslee, W. R., Gladstone, T. R., Wright, E. J., & Cooper, A. B. (2003). A family-based approach to the prevention of depressive symptoms in children at risk: Evidence of parental and child change. *Pediatrics, 112*, 119–131.

Beardslee, W. R., Wright, E. J., Salt, P., Drezner, K., Gladstone, T. R., Versage, E. M., et al. (1997). Examination of children's responses to two preventive intervention strategies over time. *Journal of the American Academy of Child and Adolescent Psychiatry, 36*, 196–204.

Becher, A., Drenckhahn, A., Pahner, I., Margittai, M., Jahn, R., & Ahnert-Hilger, G. (1999). The synaptophysin–synaptobrevin complex: A hallmark of synaptic vesicle maturation. *Journal of Neuroscience, 19*, 1922.

Beck, A. T. (1963). Thinking and depression: I. Idiosyncratic content and cognitive distortions. *Archives of General Psychiatry, 9*, 324–333.

Beck, A. T. (1967). *Depression: Causes and treatment*. Philadelphia: University of Pennsylvania Press.

Beck, A. T. (1976). *Cognitive therapy and the emotional disorders*. New York: International Universities Press.

Beck, A. T. (1983). Cognitive therapy of depression: New perspectives. In P. J. Clayton & J. E. Barret (Eds.), *Treatment of depression: Old controversies and new approaches* (pp. 265–290). New York: Raven Press.

Beck, A. T. (1987). Cognitive model of depression. *Journal of Cognitive Psychotherapy, 1*, 2–27.

Beck, A. T., & Emery, G. (1985). *Anxiety disorders and phobias: A cognitive perspective*. New York: Basic Books.

Beck, A. T., Rush, A. J., Shaw, B. F., & Emery, G. (1979). *Cognitive therapy of depression*. New York: Guilford Press.

Beckham, E. E., Leber, W. R., & Youll, L. K. (1995). The diagnostic classification of depression. In E. E. Beckham & W. R. Leber (Eds.), *Handbook of depression* (2nd ed., pp. 36–60). New York: Guilford Press.

Beevers, C. G., Ellis, A. J., Wells, T. T., & McGeary, J. E. (2010). Serotonin transporter gene promoter region polymorphism and selective processing of emotional images. *Biological Psychology, 83,* 260–265.

Beevers, C. G., Rohde, P., Stice, E., & Nolen-Hoeksema, S. (2007). Recovery from major depressive disorder among female adolescents: A prospective test of the scar hypothesis. *Journal of Consulting and Clinical Psychology, 75,* 888–900.

Beevers, C. G., Wells, T. T., Ellis, A. J., & McGeary, J. E. (2009). Association of the serotonin transporter gene promoter region (5-HTTLPR) polymorphism with biased attention for emotional stimuli. *Journal of Abnormal Psychology, 118,* 670–681.

Beevers, C. G., Wells, T. T., & McGeary, J. E. (2009). The BDNF Val66Met polymorphism is associated with rumination in healthy adults. *Emotion, 9,* 579–584.

Bemporad, J. R., & Romano, S. J. (1992). Childhood maltreatment and adult depression: A review of research. In D. Cicchetti & S. L. Toth (Eds.), *Developmental perspectives on depression.* Rochester, NY: University of Rochester Press.

Berger, M., & Riemann, D. (1993). REM-sleep in depression: An overview. *Journal of Sleep Research, 2,* 211–223.

Berman, R. M., Narasimhan, M., Sanacora, G., Miano, A. P., Hoffman, R. E., Hu, X. S., et al. (2000). A randomized clinical trial of repetitive transcranial magnetic stimulation in the treatment of major depression. *Biological Psychiatry, 47,* 332–337.

Bishop, S. R., Lau, M. A., Shapiro, S., Carlson, L., Anderson, N. D., Carmody, J., et al. (2004). Mindfulness: A proposed operational definition. *Clinical Psychology: Science and Practice, 11,* 230–241.

Billings, A. G., Cronkite, R. C., & Moos, R. H. (1983). Social–environmental factors in unipolar depression: Comparisons of depressed patients and nondepressed controls. *Journal of Abnormal Psychology, 92,* 119–133.

Billings, A. G., & Moos, R. H. (1982). Work stress and the stress-buffering roles of work and family resources. *Journal of Occupational Behavior, 3,* 215–232.

Billings, A. G., & Moos, R. H. (1983). Comparisons of children of depressed and nondepressed parents: A social–environmental perspective. *Journal of Abnormal Child Psychology, 11,* 463–485.

Billings, A. G., & Moos, R. H. (1985). Life stressors and social resources affect posttreatment outcomes among depressed patients. *Journal of Abnormal Psychology, 94,* 140–153.

Blackburn, I. M., Eunsun, K. M., & Bishop, S. (1986). A two-year naturalistic follow-up of depressed patients treated with cognitive therapy, pharmacotherapy, and a combination of both. *Journal of Affective Disorders, 10,* 67–75.

Blackburn, I. M., & Moore, R. (1997). Controlled acute and follow-up trial of cognitive therapy and pharmacotherapy in outpatients with recurrent depression. *British Journal of Psychiatry, 171,* 328–334.

Blackburn, I. M., Whalley, L. J., & Christie, J. E. (1987). Mood, cognition and cortisol: Their temporal relationships during recovery from depressive illness. *Journal of Affective Disorders, 13,* 31–43.

Blackhart, G. C., Minnix, J. A., & Kline, J. P. (2006). Can EEG asymmetry patterns predict future development of anxiety and depression?: A preliminary study. *Biological Psychology, 72,* 46–50.

Blackwood, D. H. R., Whalley, L. J., Christie, J. E., Blackburn, I. M., Stclair, D. M., & McInnes, A. (1987). Changes in auditory P3 event-related potential in schizophrenia and depression. *British Journal of Psychiatry, 150,* 154–160.

Blatt, S. J., & Homann, E. (1992). Parent–child interaction in the etiology of dependent and self-critical depression. *Clinical Psychology Review, 12,* 47–91.

Blatt, S. J., Wein, S. J., Chevron, E., & Quinlan, D. M. (1979). Parental representations and depression in normal young adults. *Journal of Abnormal Psychology, 88,* 388–397.

Blatt, S. J., & Zuroff, D. C. (1992). Interpersonal relatedness and self-definition: Two prototypes for depression. *Clinical Psychology Review, 12,* 527–562.

Bockting, C. L., Schene, A. H., Spinhoven, P., Koeter, M. W., Wouters, L. F., Huyser, J., et al. (2005). Preventing relapse/recurrence in recurrent depression with cognitive therapy: A randomized controlled trial. *Journal of Consulting and Clinical Psychology, 73,* 647–657.

Boes, A. D., McCormick, L. M., Coryell, W. H., & Nopoulos, P. (2008). Rostral anterior cingulate cortex volume correlates with depressed mood in normal healthy children. *Biological Psychiatry, 63,* 391–397.

Boland, R. J., & Keller, M. B. (2009). Course and outcome of depression. In I. Gotlib & C. Hammen (Eds.), *Handbook of depression* (2nd ed., pp. 23–43). New York: Guilford Press.

Bondolfi, G., Jermann, F., Van der Linden, M., Gex-Fabry, M., Bizzini, L., Bertschy, G., et al. (2010). Depression relapse prophylaxis with mindfulness-based cognitive therapy: Replication and extension in the Swiss health care system. *Journal of Affective Disorders, 122,* 224–231.

Boomsma, D., Vink, J., van Beijsterveldt, T., Geus, E., Beem, A., Mulder, E., et al. (2002). Netherlands Twin Register: A focus on longitudinal research. *Twin Research and Human Genetics, 5,* 401–406.

Borod, J. (1993). Cerebral mechanisms underlying facial, prosodic, and lexical emotional expression: A review of neuropsychological studies and methodological issues. *Neuropsychology, 7,* 445–463.

Borod, J. C. (2000). *The neuropsychology of emotion series in affective science.* New York: Oxford University Press.

Bowlby, J. (1961). Separation anxiety: A critical review of the literature. *Journal of Child Psychology and Psychiatry, 1,* 251–269.

Bowlby, J. (1969). *Attachment and loss: Vol. 1. Attachment.* New York: Basic Books.

Bowlby, J. (1973). *Attachment and loss: Vol. 2. Separation, anxiety, and anger.* New York: Basic Books.

Bowlby, J. (1980). *Attachment and loss: Vol. 3. Loss: Sadness and depression.* New York: Basic Books.

Bowlby, J. (1988). *A secure base: Parent–child attachment and healthy human development.* New York: Basic Books.

Boyd, J. H., Burke, J. D., Gruenberg, E., Holzer, C. E., III, Rae, D. S., George, L. K., et al. (1984). Exclusion criteria of DSM-III: A study of co-occurrence of hierarchy-free syndromes. *Archives of General Psychiatry, 41,* 983–959.

Brach, T. (2003). *Radical acceptance: Embracing your life with the heart of a Buddha.* New York: Bantam Dell.

Bradley, M., Codispoti, M., Cuthbert, B., & Lang, P. (2001). Emotion and motivation I: Defensive and appetitive reactions in picture processing. *Emotion, 1,* 276–298.

Bradley, M., & Lang, P. (2000). Measuring emotion: Behavior, feeling, and physiology. *Cognitive Neuroscience of Emotion, 25,* 49–59.

Bradley, M., & Lang, P. (2000). Measuring emotion: Behavior, feeling, and physiology. In R. Lane & L. Nadel (Eds.), *Cognitive neuroscience of emotion* (pp. 242–276). New York: Oxford University Press.

Bradley, M., Sabatinelli, D., Lang, P., Fitzsimmons, J., King, W., & Desai, P. (2003). Activation of the visual cortex in motivated attention. *Behavioral Neuroscience, 117,* 369–380.

Brandeis, D., Banaschewski, T., Baving, L., Georgiewa, P., Blanz, B., Schmidt, M. H., et al. (2002). Multicenter P300 brain mapping of impaired attention to cues in hyperkinetic children. *Journal of the American Academy of Child and Adolescent Psychiatry, 41,* 990–998.

Brefczynski-Lewis, J., Lutz, A., & Schaefer, H. (2007). Neural correlates of attentional expertise in long-term mediation practitioners. *Proceeding of the National Academy of Sciences, 104,* 11483–11488.

Bremner, J. D., Innis, R. B., Salomon, R. M., Staib, L. H., Ng, C. K., Miller, H. L., et al. (1997). Positron emission tomography measurement of cerebral metabolic correlates of tryptophan depletion-induced depressive relapse. *Archives of General Psychiatry, 54,* 364–374.

Bremner, J. D., Narayan, M., Anderson, E. R., Staib, L. H., Miller, H. L., & Charney, D. S. (2000). Hippocampal volume reduction in major depression. *American Journal of Psychiatry, 157,* 115–117.

Bremner, J. D., Vythilingam, M., Anderson, G., Vermetten, E., McGlashan, T., Heninger, G., et al. (2003). Assessment of the hypothalamic–pituitary–adrenal axis over a 24-hour diurnal period and in response to neuroendocrine challenges in women with and without childhood sexual abuse and posttraumatic stress disorder. *Biological Psychiatry, 54,* 710.

Brewin, C. R., Andrews, B., & Gotlib, I. (1993). Psychopathology and early experience: A reappraisal of retrospective reports. *Psychological Bulletin, 113,* 82–98.

Brewin, C. R., Firth-Cozens, J., Furnham, A., & McManus, C. (1992). Self-criticism in adulthood and recalled childhood experience. *Journal of Abnormal Psychology, 101*, 561–566.

Broadhead, W. E., Blazer, D. G., George, L. K., & Chiu, K. T. (1990). Depression, disability days, and days lost from work in a prospective epidemiological study. *Journal of the American Medical Association, 264*, 2524–2528.

Broderick, P. C. (2005). Mindfulness and coping with dysphoric mood: Contrasts with rumination and distraction. *Cognitive Therapy and Research, 29*, 501–510.

Brown, G. W., & Harris, T. O. (1978). *Social origins of depression: A study of psychiatric disorder in women.* London: Tavistock.

Brown, G. W., & Harris, T. O. (Eds.). (1989). *Life events and illness.* New York: Guilford Press.

Brown, K. W., & Ryan, R. M. (2006). Perils and promise in defining and measuring mindfulness: Observations from experience. *Clinical Psychology: Science and Practice, 11*, 242–248.

Brown, S. M., & Hariri, A. R. (2006). Neuroimaging studies of serotonin gene polymorphisms: Exploring the interplay of genes, brain, and behavior. *Cognitive Affective and Behavioral Neuroscience, 6*, 44–52.

Browne, A., & Finkelhor, D. (1986). Impact of child sexual abuse: A review of the research. *Psychological Bulletin, 99*, 66–77.

Bruder, G., Towey, J., Stewart, J., Friedman, D., Tenke, C., & Quitkin, F. (1991). Event-related potentials in depression: Influence of task, stimulus hemifield and clinical features on P3 latency. *Biological Psychiatry, 30*, 233–246.

Bruder, G. E., Tenke, C. E., Stewart, J. W., Towey, J. P., Leite, P., Voglmaier, M., et al. (1995). Brain event-related potentials to complex tones on depressed patients: Relations to perceptual asymmetry and clinical features. *Psychophysiology, 32*, 373–381.

Bruder, G. E., Tenke, C. E., Warner, V., Nomura, Y., Grillon, C., Hille, J., et al. (2005). Electroencephalographic measures of regional hemispheric activity in offspring at risk for depressive disorders. *Biological Psychiatry, 57*, 328–335.

Bruder, G. E., Tenke, C. E., Warner, V., & Weissman, M. M. (2007). Grandchildren at high and low risk for depression differ in EEG measures of regional brain asymmetry. *Biological Psychiatry, 62*, 1317–1323.

Burbach, D. J., & Borduin, C. M. (1986). Parent–child relations and the etiology of depression. *Clinical Psychology Review, 6*, 133–153.

Burgess, S., Geddes, J., Hawton, K., Townsend, E., Jamison, K., & Goodwin, G. (2001). Lithium for maintenance treatment of mood disorders. *Cochrane Database Systems Review, 3*, CD003013.

Calfas, K. J., Ingram, R. E., & Kaplan, R. M. (1997). Information processing and affective distress in osteoarthritis patients. *Journal of Consulting and Clinical Psychology, 65*, 576–581.

Caspi, A., Sugden, K., Moffitt, T. E., Taylor, A., Craig, I. W., Harrington, H., et al. (2003). Influence of life stress on depression: Moderation by a polymorphism in the 5-HTT gene. *Science, 301*, 386–389.

Cautela, J. R. (1970). Covert negative reinforcement. *Journal of Behavior Therapy and Experimental Psychiatry, 1*, 273–278.

Cavanagh, J., & Geisler, M. W. (2006). Mood effects on the ERP processing of emotional intensity in faces: A P3 investigation with depressed students. *International Journal of Psychophysiology, 60*, 27–33.

Chakroun, H., Bougerol, T., & Siles, S. (1988). Etude des pev et des processus attentionnels au cours de la depression. *Neurophysiologie Clinique/Clinical Neurophysiology, 18*, 161–172.

Chakroun, H., Bougerol, T., & Siles, E. (1988). Visual evoked potentials, attention process during depression. *Clinical Neurophysiology, 18*, 161–172.

Chambers, R., Lo, B. C., & Allen, N. B. (2008). The impact of intensive mindfulness training on attentional control, cognitive style and affect. *Cognitive Therapy and Research, 32*, 303–322.

Chan, S. W. Y., Harmer, C. J., Goodwin, G. M., & Norbury, R. (2008). Risk for depression is associated with neural biases in emotional categorisation. *Neuropsychologia, 46*, 2896–2903.

Chentsova-Dutton, Y. E., & Tsai, J. (2009). Understanding depression across cultures. In I. H. Gotlib & C. L. Hammen (Eds.), *Handbook of depression* (2nd ed., pp. 363–385). New York: Guilford Press.

Christensen, B. K., Carney, C. E., & Segal, Z. V. (2006). Cognitive processing models of depression. In D. J. Stein, D. J. Kupfer, & A. F. Schatzberg (Eds.), *Textbook of mood disorders* (pp. 131–144). Washington, DC: American Psychiatric Publishing.

Christensen, H., Griffiths, K. M., & Jorm, A. F. (2004). Delivering interventions for depression by using the Internet: Randomised controlled trial. *British Medical Journal, 328*, 265.

Clark, L. A. (1989). The anxiety and depressive disorders: Descriptive psychopathology and differential diagnosis. In P. C. Kendall & D. Watson (Eds.), *Anxiety and depression: Distinctive and overlapping features. Personality, psychopathology, and psychotherapy* (pp. 83–129). San Diego: Academic Press.

Clarke, G. N., Eubanks, D., Reid, E., Kelleher, C., O'Connor, E., DeBar, L. L., et al. (2005). Overcoming depression on the Internet (ODIN) (2): A randomized trial of a self-help depression skills program with reminders. *Journal of Medical Internet Research, 7*, 16.

Clarke, G. N., Hawkins, W., Murphy, M., Sheeber, L., Lewinsohn, P. M., & Seeley, J. R. (1995). Targeted prevention of unipolar depressive disorder in an at-risk sample of high school adolescents: A randomized trial of a group cognitive intervention. *Journal of the American Academy of Child and Adolescent Psychiatry, 34*, 312–321.

Clarke, G. N., Hornbrook, M., Lynch, F., Polen, M., Gale, J., Beardslee, W., et al. (2001). A randomized trial of a group cognitive intervention for preventing depression in adolescent offspring of depressed parents. *Archives of General Psychiatry, 58,* 1127–1134.

Clarke, G. N., Reid, E., Eubanks, D., O'Connor, E., DeBar, L. L., Kelleher, C., et al. (2002). Overcoming depression on the Internet (ODIN): A randomized controlled trial of an Internet depression skills intervention program. *Journal of Medical Internet Research, 4,* 14.

Coan, J. A., & Allen, J. (2004). Frontal EEG asymmetry as a moderator and mediator of emotion. *Biological Psychology, 67,* 7–50.

Coan, J. A., & Allen, J. J. B. (2003). Frontal EEG asymmetry and the behavioral activation and inhibition systems. *Psychophysiology, 40,* 106–114.

Cohen, L. (Ed.). (1988). *Research on stressful life events: Theoretical and methodological issues* (pp. 31–63). Newbury Park, CA: Sage.

Cohn, J. F., & Campbell, S. B. (1992). Influence of maternal depression on infant affect regulation. In D. Cicchetti & S. L. Toth (Eds.), *Developmental perspectives on depression* (pp. 103–130). Rochester, NY: University of Rochester Press.

Compton, R., Banich, M., Mohanty, A., Milham, M., Herrington, J., Miller, G., et al. (2003). Paying attention to emotion: An fMRI investigation of cognitive and emotional Stroop tasks. *Cognitive, Affective, and Behavioral Neuroscience, 3*(2), 81.

Corcoran, K. M., Farb, N., Anderson, A., & Segal, Z. V. (2010). Mindfulness and emotion regulation: Outcomes and possible mediating mechanisms. In A. Kring & D. Sloan (Eds.), *Emotion regulation and psychopathology* (pp. 339–355). New York: Guilford Press.

Costello, M. (2009). Age of onset. In R. E. Ingram (Ed.), *International encyclopedia of depression* (pp. 16–18). New York: Springer.

Coyne, J. C. (1976). Toward an interactional description of depression. *Psychiatry, 39,* 28–40.

Coyne, J. C., Kessler, R. C., Tal, M., Turnbull, J., Wortman, C. B., & Greden, J. F. (1987). Living with a depressed person. *Journal of Consulting and Clinical Psychology, 55,* 347–352.

Craig, A. (2002). How do you feel? Interoception: The sense of the physiological condition of the body. *Nature Reviews Neuroscience, 3,* 655–666.

Creswell, J. D., Way, B. M., Eisenberger, N. I., & Lieberman, M. D. (2007). Neural correlates of dispositional mindfulness during affect labelling. *Psychosomatic Medicine, 69,* 560–565.

Crottaz-Herbette, S., & Menon, N. (2006). Where and when the anterior cingulate cortex modulates attentional response: Combined fMRI and ERP evidence. *Journal of Cognitive Neuroscience, 18,* 766–780.

Cuijpers, P., Muñoz, R. F., Clarke, G. N., & Lewinsohn, P. M. (2009). Psychoeducational treatment and prevention of depression: The "Coping with Depression" course thirty years later. *Clinical Psychology Review, 29,* 449–458.

Cummings, E. M., & Cicchetti, D. (1990). Toward a transactional model of relations between attachment and depression. In M. Greenberg & D. Cicchetti (Eds.), *Attachment in the preschool years: Theory, research, and intervention* (pp. 339–372). Chicago: University of Chicago Press.

Cuthbert, B., Lang, P., Strauss, C., Drobes, D., Patrick, C., & Bradley, M. (2003). The psychophysiology of anxiety disorder: Fear memory imagery. *Psychophysiology, 40*, 407–422.

Cutler, S. E., & Nolen-Hoeksema, S. (1991). Accounting for sex differences in depression through female victimization: Childhood sexual abuse. *Sex Roles, 24*, 425–438.

Daffner, K., Mesulam, M., Scinto, L., Acar, D., Calvo, V., Faust, R., et al. (2000). The central role of the prefrontal cortex in directing attention to novel events. *Brain, 123*, 927.

Damasio, A. (1998). Emotion in the perspective of an integrated nervous system. *Brain Research Reviews, 26*, 83–86.

Damasio, A., Grabowski, T., Bechara, A., Damasio, H., Ponto, L., Parvizi, J., et al. (2000). Subcortical and cortical brain activity during the feeling of self-generated emotions. *Nature Neuroscience, 3*, 1049–1056.

Davidson, R. (1992). Emotion and affective style: Hemispheric substrates. *Psychological Science, 3*, 39.

Davidson, R. (1993). Parsing affective space: Perspectives from neuropsychology and psychophysiology. *Neuropsychology, 7*, 464–475.

Davidson, R. (1994). On emotion, mood, and related affective constructs. In P. Ekman & R. J. Davidson (Eds.), *The nature of emotion: Fundamental questions* (pp. 51–55). New York: Oxford University Press.

Davidson, R. (1998). Anterior electrophysiological asymmetries, emotion, and depression: Conceptual and methodological conundrums. *Psychophysiology, 35*, 607–614.

Davidson, R. (2000). Affective style, psychopathology, and resilience: Brain mechanisms and plasticity. *American Psychologist, 55*, 1196–1214.

Davidson, R. (2001). Toward a biology of personality and emotion. *Annals of the New York Academy of Sciences, 935*, 191–207.

Davidson, R. (2002). Anxiety and affective style: Role of prefrontal cortex and amygdala. *Biological Psychiatry, 51*, 68–80.

Davidson, R. (2003). Affective neuroscience and psychophysiology: Toward a synthesis. *Psychophysiology, 40*, 655–665.

Davidson, R., Ekman, P., Saron, C., Senulis, J., & Friesen, W. (1990). Approach-withdrawal and cerebral asymmetry: Emotional expression and brain physiology I. *Journal of Personality and Social Psychology, 58* 330–341.

Davidson, R., & Fox, N. (1989). Frontal brain asymmetry predicts infants' response to maternal separation. *Journal of Abnormal Psychology, 98*, 127–131.

Davidson, R., & Irwin, W. (1999). The functional neuroanatomy of emotion and affective style. *Trends in Cognitive Sciences, 3*, 11–21.

Davidson, R., Jackson, D., & Kalin, N. (2000). Emotion, plasticity, context, and regulation: Perspectives from affective neuroscience. *Psychological Bulletin, 126*, 890–909.

Davidson, R., Pizzagalli, D., & Nitschke, J. B. (2002). The representation and regulation of emotion in depression: Perspectives from affective neuroscience. In I. H. Gotlib & C. L. Hammen (Eds.), *Handbook of depression* (pp. 219–244). New York: Guilford Press.

Davidson, R., Pizzagalli, D., Nitschke, J., & Putnam, K. (2002). Depression: Perspectives from affective neuroscience. *Annual Review of Psychology, 53*, 545–574.

Davidson, R., Putnam, K., & Larson, C. (2000). Dysfunction in the neural circuitry of emotion regulation—a possible prelude to violence. *Science, 289*, 591.

Davidson, R., Schaffer, C., & Saron, C. (1985). Effects of lateralized presentations of faces on self-reports of emotion and EEG asymmetry in depressed and nondepressed subjects. *Psychophysiology, 22*, 353–363.

Dawson, G., Frey, K., Panagiotides, H., Osterling, J., & Hessl, D. (2006). Infants of depressed mothers exhibit atypical frontal brain activity: A replication and extension of previous findings. *Journal of Child Psychology and Psychiatry, 38*, 179–186.

Dawson, G., Frey, K., Panagiotides, H., Yamada, E., Hessl, D., & Osterling, J. (1999). Infants of depressed mothers exhibit atypical frontal electrical brain activity during interactions with mother and with a familiar, nondepressed adult. *Child Development, 70*, 1058–1066.

Dawson, G., Klinger, L. G., Panagiotides, H., Hill, D., & Spieker, S. (1992). Frontal lobe activity and affective behavior of infants of mothers with depressive symptoms. *Child Development, 63*, 725–737.

Dawson, G., Panagiotides, H., Klinger, L., & Spieker, S. (1997). Infants of depressed and nondepressed mothers exhibit differences in frontal brain electrical activity during the expression of negative emotions. *Developmental Psychology, 33*, 650–656.

Dearing, K. F., & Gotlib, I. H. (2009). Interpretation of ambiguous information in girls at risk for depression. *Journal of Abnormal Child Psychology, 37*, 79–91.

de Geus, E. J. C., van't Ent, D., Wolfensberger, S. P. A., Heutink, P., Hoogendijk, W. J. G., Boomsma, D. I., et al. (2007). Intrapair differences in hippocampal volume in monozygotic twins discordant for the risk for anxiety and depression. *Biological Psychiatry, 61*, 1062–1071.

Demyttenaere, K., Enzlin, P., Dewe, W., Boulinger, B., De Bie, J., De Troyer, E., et al. (2001). Compliance with antidepressants in a primary care setting: Beyond lack of efficacy and adverse events. *Journal of Clinical Psychiatry, 62*(Suppl.), 30–33.

Dennett, D. (1991). *Consciousness Explained.* New York: Little, Brown & Co.

Dent, J., & Teasdale, J. D. (1988). Negative cognition and the persistence of depression. *Journal of Abnormal Psychology, 97*, 29–34.

Depression Guideline Panel. (1993). *Depression in primary care: Vol. 2. Treatment of major depression. Clinical practice guideline, Number 5* (AHCPR Pub. No. 93-0551). Rockville, MD: U.S. Department of Health and

Human Services, Public Health Service, Agency for Health Care Policy and Research.

Depue, R. A., & Iacono, W. G. (1989). Neurobehavioral aspects of affective disorders. *Annual Review of Psychology, 40*, 457–492.

Depue, R. A., & Kleiman, R. M. (1979). Free cortisol as a perpheral index of central vulnerability to major forms of unipolar depressive disorders: Examining stress–biology interactions in subsyndromal high risk persons. In R. A. Depue (Ed.), *The psychobiology of depressive disorders* (pp. 177–204). New York: Academic Press.

Depue, R. A., Kleiman, R. M., Davis, P., Hutchinson, M., & Krauss, S. (1985). The behavioral high-risk paradigm and bipolar affective disorder: VIII. Serum free cortisol in nonpatient cyclothymic subjects selected by the General Behavior Inventory. *American Journal of Psychiatry, 142*, 175–181.

Depue, R. A., Krauss, S., Spoont, M., & Arbisi, P. (1989). Identification of unipolar and bipolar affective conditions in a university population with the General Behavior Inventory. *Journal of Abnormal Psychology, 98*, 117–126.

Depue, R. A., & Monroe, S. M. (1986). Conceptualization and measurement of human disorder and life stress research: The problem of chronic disturbance. *Psychological Bulletin, 85*, 1001–1029.

Depue, R. A., Slater, J. F., Wolfstetter-Kausch, H., Klein, D., Goplerud, E., & Farr, D. (1981). A behavioral paradigm for identifying persons at risk for bipolar depressive disorder: A conceptual framework and five validation studies. *Journal of Abnormal Psychology, 90*, 381–437.

Derryberry, D., & Tucker, D. (1992). Neural mechanisms of emotion. *Journal of Consulting and Clinical Psychology, 60*, 329–338.

DeRubeis, R. J., Evans, M. D., & Hollon, S. D. (1990). How does cognitive therapy work?: Cognitive change and symptom change in cognitive therapy and pharmacotherapy for depression. *Journal of Consulting and Clinical Psychology, 6*, 862–869.

DeRubeis, R. J., Siegle, G. J., & Hollon, S. D. (2008). Cognitive therapy versus medication for depression: Treatment outcomes and neural mechanisms. *Nature Reviews: Neuroscience, 9*, 788–796.

Devinsky, O., Morrell, M. J., & Vogt, B. A. (1995). Contributions of anterior cingulated cortex to behaviour. *Brain, 118*, 279–306.

Diner, B. C., Holcomb, P. J., & Dykman, R. A. (1985). P300 in major depressive disorder. *Psychiatry Research, 15*, 175–184.

Doane, J. A., & Diamond, D. (1994). *Affect and attachment in the family: A family based treatment of major psychiatric disorder.* New York: Basic Books.

Dobson, K., & Shaw, B. (1986). Cognitive assessment with major depressive disorders. *Cognitive Therapy and Research, 10*, 13–29.

Dobson, K., & Shaw, B. (1987). Specificity and stability of self-referent encoding in clinical depression. *Journal of Abnormal Psychology, 96*, 34–40.

Dodge, K. A. (1993). Social-cognitive mechanisms in the development of conduct disorder and depression. *Annual Review of Psychology, 44,* 559–584.

Dohrenwend, B. P., & Shrout, P. E. (1985). "Hassles" in the conceptualization and measurement of life stress variables. *American Psychologist, 40,* 780–785.

Donders, F. C. (1969). Over de snelheid van psychische processen. Onderzoekingen gedaan in het Physiologisch Laboratorium der Utrechtsche Hoogeschool, 1868–1869, Tweede reeks II, 92–120. Translated by W. G. Koster in W. G. Koster (Ed.), *Attention and performance: II. Acta Psychologica, 30,* 412–431.

Dorzab, J., Baker, M., Winokur, G., & Cadoret, R. J. (1971). Depressive disease: Clinical course. *Diseases of the Nervous System, 32,* 269–273.

Downey, G., & Coyne, J. C. (1990). Children of depressed parents: An integrative review. *Psychological Bulletin, 108,* 50–75.

Drevets, W. (1999). Prefrontal cortical-amygdalar metabolism in major depression. *Annals of the New York Academy of Sciences, 877,* 614–637.

Drevets, W., Price, J., Todd, R., Reich, T., Bardgett, M., Csernansky, J., et al. (1997). PET measures of amygdala metabolism in bipolar and unipolar depression: Correlation with plasma cortisol. *Society of Neuroscience Abstract, 23,* 1407.

Drevets, W. C. (1998). Functional neuroimaging studies of depression: The anatomy of melancholia. *Annual Review of Medicine, 49,* 341–361.

Drevets, W. C. (2000). Neuroimaging studies of mood disorders. *Biological Psychiatry, 48,* 813–829.

Drevets, W. C. (2008). Neuroplasticity, neuroimaging and depression. *International Journal of Neuropsychopharmacology, 11,* 41–41.

Drevets, W. C., Price, J., Bardgett, M., Reich, T., Todd, R., & Raichle, M. (2002). Glucose metabolism in the amygdala in depression: Relationship to diagnostic subtype and plasma cortisol levels. *Pharmacology Biochemistry and Behavior, 71,* 431–448.

Drevets, W. C., Price, J. L., & Furey, M. L. (2008). Brain structural and functional abnormalities in mood disorders: Implications for neurocircuitry models of depression. *Brain Structure and Function, 213,* 93–118.

Drevets, W. C., Price, J., Simpson, J., Todd, R., Reich, T., Vannier, M., et al. (1997). Subgenual prefrontal cortex abnormalities in mood disorders. *Nature, 386,* 824–827.

Drevets, W. C., Videen, T., Price, J., Preskorn, S., Carmichael, S., & Raichle, M. (1992). A functional anatomical study of unipolar depression. *Journal of Neuroscience, 12,* 3628.

Dryman, A., & Eaton, W. W. (1991). Affective symptoms associated with the onset of major depression in the community: Findings from the U.S. National Institute of Mental Health Epidemiological Catchment Area Program. *Acta Psychiatrica Scandinavica, 84,* 1–5.

Dubal, S., Pierson, A., & Jouvent, R. (2000). Focused attention in anhedonia: A P3 study. *Psychophysiology, 37,* 711–714.

Dunkley, D. M., Sanislow, C. A., Grilo, C. M., & McGlashan, T. H. (2009). Self-criticism versus neuroticism in predicting depression and psychosocial impairment for 4 years in a clinical sample. *Comprehensive Psychiatry, 50,* 335–346.

Dykman, B. M. (1997). A test of whether negative emotional priming facilitates access to latent dysfunctional attitudes. *Cognition and Emotion, 11,* 197–222.

Eaton, W. W., Holzer, C. E., Von Korff, Anthony, J. C., Helzer, J. E., George, L., et al. (1984). The design of the Epidemiologic Catchment Area surveys: The control and measurement of error. *Archives of General Psychiatry, 41,* 942–948.

Eaton, W. W., & Kessler, L. G. (Eds.). (1985). *Epidemiologic field methods in psychiatry: The NIMH Epidemiologic Catchment Area Program.* New York: Academic Press.

Eberhart, N. K., & Hammen, C. L. (2009). Interpersonal predictors of stress generation. *Personality and Social Psychology Bulletin, 35,* 544–556.

Elkin, I., Shea, M. T., Watkins, J. T., Imber, S. D., Sotsky, S. M., Collins, J. F., et al. (1989). National Institute of Mental Health Treatment of Depression Collaborative Research Program: General effectiveness of treatments. *Archives of General Psychiatry, 46,* 971–982.

Ellis, A. (1962). *Reason and emotion in psychotherapy.* New York: Lyle Stuart.

Engel, R. A., & DeRubeis, R. J. (1993). The role of cognition in depression. In K. S. Dobson & P. C. Kendall (Eds.), *Psychopathology and cognition* (pp. 83–119). San Diego: Academic Press.

Epstein, J., Pan, H., Kocsis, J., Yang, Y., Butler, T., Chusid, J., et al. (2006). Lack of ventral striatal response to positive stimuli in depressed versus normal subjects. *American Journal of Psychiatry, 163,* 1784.

Eriksen, C., & Yeh. (1985). Allocation of attention in the visual field. *Journal of Experimental Psychology: Human Perception and Performance, 11,* 583–597.

Evans, M. D., Hollon, S. D., DeRubeis, R. J., Piasecki, J. M., Grove, W. M., Garvey, M. J., et al. (1992). Differential relapse following cognitive therapy and pharmacotherapy for depression. *Archives of General Psychiatry, 49,* 802–808.

Eysenck, S., Eysenck, H., & Barrett, P. (1985). A revised version of the Psychoticism Scale. *Personality and Individual Differences, 6,* 21–29.

Fales, C., Barch, D., Rundle, M., Mintun, M., Snyder, A., Cohen, J., et al. (2008). Altered emotional interference processing in affective and cognitive-control brain circuitry in major depression. *Biological Psychiatry, 63*(4), 377–384.

Farb, N., Segal, Z. V., Mayberg, H., Bean, J., McKeon, D., Fatima, Z., et al. (2007). Attending to the present: Mindfulness meditation reveals distinct neural modes of self-reference. *Social Cognitive and Affective Neuroscience, 2,* 313–322.

Farb, N. A., Anderson, A. K., Corcoran, K., Bloch, R., Bean, J., McKeon, D., et al. (2010). *Comparing the effects of relaxation or mindfulness on neural markers of emotion regulation.* Manuscript under review

Farb, N. A., Anderson, A. K., Mayberg, H., Bean, J., McKeon, D., & Segal Z. V. (2010). Minding one's emotions: Mindfulness training alters the neural expression of sadness. *Emotion, 10,* 25–33. (Erratum in: *Emotion,* 2010, *10,* 215.)

Farb, N. A., Anderson, A. K., & Segal, Z. V. (2010). *Neural correlates of sadness reactivity and prediction of relapse outcomes in recovered depressed patients at 18 months.* Manuscript under review.

Fava, G. A., Grandi, S., Zielezny, M., Rafanelli, C., & Canestrari, R. (1996). Four-year outcome for cognitive behavioural treatment of residual symptoms in primary major depressive disorder. *American Journal of Psychiatry, 153,* 945–947.

Fava, G. A., Rafanelli, C., Grandi, S., Conti, S., & Belluardo, P. (1998). Prevention of recurrent depression with cognitive behavioral therapy: Preliminary findings. *Archives of General Psychiatry, 55,* 816–820.

Fava, G. A., Ruini, C., & Rafanelli, C. (2005). Sequential treatment of mood and anxiety disorders. *Journal of Clinical Psychiatry, 66,* 1392–1400.

Fava, G. A., Tomba, E., & Grandi, S. (2007). The road to recovery from depression: Don't drive today with yesterday's map. *Psychotherapy and Psychosomatics, 76,* 260–265.

Feng, J., Yan, Z., Ferreira, A., Tomizawa, K., Liauw, J. A., Zhuo, M., et al. (2000). Spinophilin regulates the formation and function of dendritic spines. *Proceedings of the National Academy of Sciences of the United States of America, 97,* 9287–9292.

Fennell, M. J. V., & Campbell, E. A. (1984). The Cognitions Questionnaire: Specific thinking errors in depression. *British Journal of Clinical Psychology, 23,* 81–92.

Field, T. (1992). Infants of depressed mothers. *Development and Psychopathology, 4,* 49–66.

Field, T. (1998). Maternal depression effects on infants and early interventions. *Preventive Medicine, 27,* 200.

Field, T. (2000). Infants of depressed mothers. In S. L. Johnson, A. M. Hayes, T. M. Field, N. Schneiderman, & P. M. McCabe (Eds.), *Stress, coping and depression* (pp. 3–22). Mahwah, NJ: Erlbaum.

Field, T. (2002). Violence and touch deprivation in adolescents. *Adolescence, 37,* 735–749.

Field, T., Diego, M., & Hernandez-Reif, M. (2006). Prenatal depression effects on the fetus and newborn: A review. *Infant Behavior and Development, 29,* 445–455.

Field, T., Fox, N., Pickens, J., & Nawrocki, T. (1995). Relative right frontal EEG activation in 3-to 6-month-old infants of "depressed" mothers. *Developmental Psychology, 31,* 358–363.

Finger, S. (1994). History of neuropsychology. In D. W. Zaidel (Ed.), *Neuropsy-*

chology: Handbook of perception and cognition (2nd ed., pp. 1–28). San Diego: Academic Press.

Frank, E., Kupfer, D. J., Jacob, M., & Jarrett, D. (1987). Personality features and response to acute treatment in recurrent depression. *Journal of Personality Disorders, 1,* 14–26.

Frank, E., Kupfer, D. J., Perel, J. M., Cornes, C., Jarrett, D. B., Mallinger, A. G., et al. (1990). Three year outcomes for maintenance therapies in recurrent depression. *Archives of General Psychiatry, 47,* 1093–1099.

Frank, E., Prien, R. F., Jarret, R. B., Keller, M. B., Kupfer, D. J., Lavori, P. W., et al. (1991). Conceptualization and rationale for consensus definitions of terms in major depressive disorder: Remission, recovery, relapse, and recurrence. *Archives of General Psychiatry, 48,* 851–855.

Fredman, L., Weissman, M. M., Leaf, P. J., & Bruce, M. L. (1988). Social functioning in community residents with depression and other psychiatric disorders: Results of the New Haven Epidemiologic Catchment Area study. *Journal of Affective Disorders, 15,* 103–112.

Freedland, K., & Carney, R. (2009). Depression and medical illness. In I. H. Gotlib & C. L. Hammen (Eds.), *Handbook of Depression* (2nd ed., pp. 113–141). New York: Guilford Press.

Fresco, D. M., Moore, M. T., van Dulmen, M. H., Segal, Z. V., Ma, S. H., Teasdale, J. D., et al. (2007). Initial psychometric properties of the Experiences Questionnaire: Validation of a self-report measure of decentering. *Behavior Therapy, 38,* 234–246.

Fresco, D. M., Segal, Z. V., Buis, T., & Kennedy, S. (2007). Relationship of post-treatment decentering and cognitive reactivity to relapse in major depression. *Journal of Consulting and Clinical Psychology, 75,* 447–455.

Frewen, P. A., Evans, E. M., Maraj, N., Dozois, D. J., & Partridge, K. (2008). Letting go: Mindfulness and negative automatic thinking. *Cognitive Therapy and Research, 32,* 758–774.

Friess, E., Modell, S., Brunner, H., Tagaya, H., Lauer, C. J., Holsboer, F., et al. (2008). The Munich vulnerability study on affective disorders: Microstructure of sleep in high-risk subjects. *European Archives of Psychiatry and Clinical Neuroscience, 258,* 285–291.

Frijda, N. (1986). *The emotions.* Cambridge: Cambridge University Press.

Frodl, T., Meisenzahl, E. M., Zetzsche, T., Born, C., Groll, C., Jager, M., et al. (2002). Hippocampal changes in patients with a first episode of major depression. *American Journal of Psychiatry, 159,* 1112–1118.

Frodl, T., Moller, H. J., & Meisenzahl, E. (2008). Neuroimaging genetics: New perspectives in research on major depression? *Acta Psychiatrica Scandinavica, 118,* 363–372.

Fuster, J. M. (1997). Network memory. *Trends in Neurosciences, 20,* 451–459.

Fuster, J. M. (2001). The prefrontal cortex—An update: Time is of the essence. *Neuron, 30,* 319–333.

Gainotti, G. (1972). Emotional behavior and hemispheric side of the lesion. *Cortex, 8,* 41–55.

Garber, J. (2008). Prevention of depression: Are we there yet? *Clinical Psychology: Science and Practice, 15*, 336–341.

Garber, J. (2010). Vulnerability to depression in childhood and adolescence. In R. E. Ingram & J. M. Price (Eds.), *Vulnerability to psychopathology: Risk across the lifespan* (2nd ed., pp. 189–247). New York: Guilford Press.

Garber, J., Clarke, G. N., Weersing, V. R., Beardslee, W. R., Brent, D. A., Gladstone, T. R., et al. (2009). Prevention of depression in at-risk adolescents: A randomized controlled trial. *Journal of the American Medical Association, 301*, 2215–2224.

Garber, J., Gallerani, C. M., & Frankal, S. A. (2009). Depression in children. In I. H. Gotlib & C. L. Hammen (Eds.), *Handbook of depression* (2nd ed., pp. 405–443). New York: Guilford Press.

Garber, J., & Hollon, S. D. (1991). What can specificity designs say about causality in psychopathology research? *Psychological Bulletin, 110*, 129–136.

Garber, J., & Robinson, N. S. (1997). Cognitive vulnerability in children at risk for depression. *Cognition and Emotion, 11*, 619–635.

Garmezy, N., & Devine, V. (1984). Project competence: The Minnesota studies of children vulnerable to psychopathology. In N. Watt, E. J. Anthony, L. Wynne, & J. Rolf (Eds.), *Children at risk for schizophrenia* (pp. 289–303). New York: Cambridge University Press.

Garratt, G., Ingram, R. E., Rand, K. L., & Sawalani, G. (2007). Cognitive processes in cognitive therapy: Evaluation of the mechanisms of change in the treatment of depression. *Clinical Psychology: Science and Practice, 14*, 224–239.

Garrison, C. Z., Addy, C. L., Jackson, K. L., McKeown, R. E., & Waller, J. L. (1992). Major depressive disorder and dysthymia in young adolescents. *American Journal of Epidemiology, 135*, 792–802.

Gelfand, D. M., & Teti, D. M. (1990). The effects of maternal depression on children. *Clinical Psychology Review, 10*, 329–353.

Gemar, M., Segal, Z. V., Sagrati, S., & Kennedy, S. (2001). Mood-induced changes on the Implicit Association Test in recovered depressed patients. *Journal of Abnormal Psychology, 110*, 282–289.

Gemar, M. C., Segal, Z. V., Mayberg, H. S., Goldapple, K., & Carney, C. (2007). Changes in regional cerebral blood flow following mood challenge in drug-free, remitted patients with unipolar depression. *Depression and Anxiety, 24*, 597–601.

George, M. S., Ketter, T. A., Parekh, P. I., Rosinsky, N., Ring, H. A., Pazzaglia, P. J., et al. (1997). Blunted left cingulate activation in mood disorder subjects during a response interference task (the Stroop). *Journal of Neuropsychiatry and Clinical Neurosciences, 9*, 55–63.

Gerlsma, C., Emmelkamp, P. M. G., & Arrindell, W. A. (1990). Anxiety, depression, and perception of early parenting: A meta-analysis. *Clinical Psychology Review, 10*, 251–277.

Germer, C. K., Siegel, R. D., & Fulton, P. R. (2005). *Mindfulness and psychotherapy*. New York: Guilford Press.

Gilbertson, M. W., Shenton, M. E., Ciszewski, A., Kasai, K., Lasko, N. B., Orr, S. P., et al. (2002). Smaller hippocampal volume predicts pathologic vulnerability to psychological trauma. *Nature Neuroscience, 5,* 1242–1247.

Gilboa, E., & Gotlib, I. (1997). Cognitive biases and affect persistence in previously dysphoric and never-dysphoric individuals. *Cognition and Emotion, 11,* 517–538.

Giles, D., Kupfer, D., Rush, A., & Roffwarg, H. (1998). Controlled comparison of electrophysiological sleep in families of probands with unipolar depression. *American Journal of Psychiatry, 155,* 192–199.

Gillham, J. E., Reivich, K. J., Freres, D. R., Lascher, M., Litzinger, S., Shatte, A., et al. (2006). School-based prevention of depression and anxiety symptoms in early adolescence: A pilot of a parent intervention component. *School Psychology Quarterly, 21,* 323–348.

Gillham, J. E., Reivich, K. J., Jaycox, L. H., & Seligman, M. E. (1995). Prevention of depressive symptoms in school children: Two-year follow-up. *Psychological Science, 6,* 343–351.

Gladstone, T. R., & Kaslow, N. J. (1995). Depression and attributions in children and adolescents: A meta-analytic review. *Journal of Abnormal Child Psychology, 23,* 597–606.

Glen, A. I., Johnson, A. L., & Shepherd, M. (1984). Continuation therapy with lithium and amitriptyline in unipolar depressive illness: A randomized, double blind, controlled trial. *Psychological Medicine, 14,* 37–50.

Goldapple, K., Segal, Z., Garson, C., Lau, M., Bieling, P., Kennedy, S., et al. (2004). Modulation of cortical–limbic pathways in major depression: Treatment-specific effects of cognitive behavior therapy. *Archives of General Psychiatry, 61,* 34–41.

Goldin, P., McRae, K., Ramel, W., & Gross, J. (2008). The neural bases of emotion regulation: Reappraisal and suppression of negative emotion. *Biological Psychiatry, 63,* 577–586.

Goodman, S., & Gotlib, I. H. (2002). Transmission of risk to children of depressed parents: Integration and conclusions. In S. Goodman & I. Gotlib (Eds.), *Children of depressed parents: Mechanisms of risk and implications for treatment* (pp. 307–326). Washington: American Psychological Association.

Goodman, S. H. (2007). Depression in mothers. *Annual Review of Clinical Psychology, 3,* 107–135.

Goodman, S. H., & Brand, S. R. (2009). Depression and early adversity. In I. H. Gotlib & C. L. Hammen (Eds.), *Handbook of depression* (2nd ed., pp. 249–274). New York: Guilford Press.

Goodman, S. H., & Tully, E. (2008). Children of depressed mothers: Implications for the etiology, treatment, and prevention of depression in children and adolescents. In J. Abela & B. Hankin (Eds.), *Handbook of depression in children and adolescents* (pp. 415–440). New York: Guilford Press.

Goodnick, P. J., & Goldstein, B. J. (1998). Selective serotonin reuptake inhibitors in affective disorders: I. Basic pharmacology. *Journal of Psychopharmacology, 12,* 5–20.

Gotlib, I., Hamilton, J., Cooney, R., Singh, M., Henry, M., & Joormann, J. (2010). Neural processing of reward and loss in girls at risk for major depression. *Archives of General Psychiatry, 67,* 380.

Gotlib, I., McLachlan, A., & Katz, N. (1988). Biases in visual attention in depressed and nondepressed individuals. *Cognition and Emotion, 2,* 185–200.

Gottesman, I. I., & Shields, J. (1972). *Schizophrenia and genetics.* New York: Academic Press.

Greenberg, L. S., Ford, C. L., Alden, L. S., & Johnson, S. M. (1993). In-session change in emotionally focused therapy. *Journal of Consulting and Clinical Psychology, 61,* 78–84.

Greil, W., Ludwig-Mayerhofer, W., Erazo, N., Engel, R., Czernik, A., Giedke, H., et al. (1996). Comparative efficacy of lithium and amitriptyline in the maintenance treatment of recurrent unipolar depression: A randomized study. *Journal of Affective Disorders, 40,* 179–190.

Grepmair, L., Mitterlehner, F., Loew, T., Bachler, E., Rother, W., & Nickel M. (2007). Promoting mindfulness in psychotherapists in training influences the treatment results of their patients: A randomized, double-blind, controlled study. *Psychotherapy and Psychosomatics, 76,* 332–338.

Grillon, C., Warner, V., Hille, J., Merikangas, K. R., Bruder, G. E., Tenke, C. E., et al. (2005). Families at high and low risk for depression: A three-generation startle study. *Biological Psychiatry, 57,* 953–960.

Gross, J. (2002). Emotion regulation: Affective, cognitive, and social consequences. *Psychophysiology, 39,* 281–291.

Guhtrie, E. R. (1935). *Psychology of learning.* New York: Harper.

Haaga, D. F., Dyck, M. J., & Ernst, D. (1991). Empirical status of cognitive theory of depression. *Psychological Bulletin, 110,* 215–236.

Haaga, D. F., & Solomon, A. (1993). Impact of Kendall, Hollon, Beck, Hammen, and Ingram (1987) on treatment of the continuity issue in "depression" research. *Cognitive Therapy and Research, 17,* 313–324.

Hajek, T., Kozeny, J., Kopecek, M., Alda, M., & Hoschl, C. (2008). Reduced subgenual cingulate volumes in mood disorders: A meta-analysis. *Journal of Psychiatry and Neuroscience, 33,* 91–99.

Haldane, M., Jogia, J., Cobb, A., Kozuch, E., Kumari, V., & Frangou, S. (2008). Changes in brain activation during working memory and facial recognition tasks in patients with bipolar disorder with Lamotrigine monotherapy. *European Neuropsychopharmacology, 18,* 48.

Hamilton, E. W., & Abramson, L. Y. (1983). Cognitive patterns and major depressive disorder: A longitudinal study in a hospital study. *Journal of Abnormal Psychology, 92,* 173–184.

Hamilton, J. P., Siemer, M., & Gotlib, I. H. (2008). Amygdala volume in major depressive disorder: A meta-analysis of magnetic resonance imaging studies. *Molecular Psychiatry, 13,* 993–1000.

Hammen, C. L. (1991). *Depression runs in families: The social context of risk and resilience in children of depressed mothers.* New York: Springer-Verlag.

Hammen, C. L. (1992). Life events and depression: The plot thickens. *American Journal of Community Psychology, 20,* 179–193.

Hammen, C. L. (2009). Children of depressed parents. In I. H. Gotlib & C. L. Hammen (Eds.), *Handbook of depression* (2nd ed., pp. 275–297). New York: Guilford Press.

Hanh, T. N. (1976). *The miracle of mindfulness: A manual for meditation.* Boston: Beacon Press.

Hankin, B. L. (2005). Childhood maltreatment and psychopathology: Prospective tests of attachment, cognitive vulnerability, and stress as mediating processes. *Cognitive Therapy and Research, 29,* 645–671.

Hariri, A. R., Mattay, V. S., Tessitore, A., Kolachana, B., Fera, F., Goldman, D., et al. (2002). Serotonin transporter genetic variation and the response of the human amygdala. *Science, 297,* 400–403.

Harvey, P., Pruessner, J., Czechowska, Y., & Lepage, M. (2007). Individual differences in trait anhedonia: A structural and functional magnetic resonance imaging study in non-clinical subjects. *Molecular Psychiatry, 12,* 767–775.

Hautzinger, M., & Bailer, M. (1993). *Allgemeine Depressions-Skala.* Weinheim: Beltz Test.

Hawley, L. L., Ho, M. H., Zuroff, D. C., & Blatt, S. J. (2006). The relationship of perfectionism, depression, and therapeutic alliance during treatment for depression: Latent difference score analysis. *Journal of Consulting and Clinical Psychology, 74,* 930–942.

Hayden, E. P., Shankman, S. A., Olino, T. M., Durbin, C. E., Tenke, C. E., Bruder, G. E., et al. (2008). Cognitive and temperamental vulnerability to depression: Longitudinal associations with regional cortical activity. *Cognition and Emotion, 22,* 1415–1428.

Hayes, S. C., & Feldman, G. (2004). Clarifying the construct of mindfulness in the context of emotion regulation and the process of change in therapy. *Clinical Psychology: Science and Practice, 11,* 255–262.

Hayes, S. C., Strosahl, K., & Willson, K. G. (1999). *Acceptance and commitment therapy: An experiential approach to behavior change.* New York: Guilford Press.

Hedlund, S., & Rude, S. S. (1995). Evidence of latent depressive schemas in formerly depressed individuals. *Journal of Abnormal Psychology, 104,* 517–525.

Heller, A., Johnstone, T., Shackman, A., Light, S., Peterson, M., Kolden, G., et al. (2009). Reduced capacity to sustain positive emotion in major depression reflects diminished maintenance of fronto-striatal brain activation. *Proceedings of the National Academy of Sciences, 106,* 22445.

Heller, W. (1993). Gender differences in depression: Perspectives from neuropsychology. *Journal of Affective Disorders, 29,* 129–143.

Heller, W. (1993). Neuropsychological mechanisms of individual differences in emotion, personality, and arousal. *Neuropsychology, 7*, 476–489.

Heller, W., & Nitschke, J. (1997). Regional brain activity in emotion: A framework for understanding cognition in depression. *Cognition and Emotion, 11*, 637–662.

Heller, W., Nitschke, J., & Miller, G. (1998). Lateralization in emotion and emotional disorders. *Current Directions in Psychological Science, 7*, 26–32.

Hendren, R. I. (1983). Depression in anorexia nervosa. *Journal of the American Academy of Child Psychiatry, 22*, 59–62.

Henriques, J., & Davidson, R. (1991). Left frontal hypoactivation in depression. *Journal of Abnormal Psychology, 100*, 535–545.

Hochstrasser, B., Isaksen, P., Koponen, H., Lauritzen, L., Mahnert, F., Rouillon, F., et al. (2001). Prophylactic effect of citalopram in unipolar recurrent depression: Placebo-controlled study of maintenance therapy. *British Journal of Psychiatry, 178*, 304–310.

Hollon, S. D. (1992). Cognitive models of depression from a psychobiological perspective. *Psychological Inquiry, 3*, 250–253.

Hollon, S. D., & Cobb, R. (1993). Relapse and recurrence in psychopathological disorders. In C. G. Costello (Ed.), *Basic issues in psychopathology* (pp. 377–402). New York: Guilford Press.

Hollon, S. D., DeRubeis, R. J., Shelton, R. C., Amsterdam, J. D., Salomon, R. M., O'Reardon, J. P., et al. (2005). Prevention of relapse following cognitive therapy vs. medications in moderate to severe depression. *Archives of General Psychiatry, 62*, 417–422.

Hollon, S. D., Evans, M. D., & DeRubeis, R. J. (1990). Cognitive mediation of relapse prevention following treatment for depression: Implications of differential risk. In R. E. Ingram (Ed.), *Contemporary psychological approaches to depression: Theory, research, and treatment* (pp. 117–136). New York: Plenum Press.

Hollon, S. D., & Kendall, P. C. (1980). Cognitive self-statements in depression: Development of an automatic thoughts questionnaire. *Cognitive Therapy and Research, 4*, 383–395.

Hollon, S. D., Stewart, M. O., & Strunk, D. R. (2006). Enduring effects for cognitive behavior therapy in the treatment of depression and anxiety. *Annual Review of Psychology, 57*, 285–315.

Hooley, J., Gruber, S., Parker, H., Guillaumot, J., Rogowska, J., & Yurgelun-Todd, D. (2009). Cortico-limbic response to personally challenging emotional stimuli after complete recovery from depression. *Psychiatry Research: Neuroimaging, 172*, 83–91.

Horowitz, M. J. (1988). *Introduction to psychodynamics: A synthesis.* New York: Basic Books.

Ilardi, S., Atchley, R., Enloe, A., Kwasny, K., & Garratt, G. (2007). Disentangling attentional biases and attentional deficits in depression: An event-related potential P300 analysis. *Cognitive Therapy and Research, 31*, 175–187.

Ingram, R. E. (1984). Toward an information processing analysis of depression. *Cognitive Therapy and Research, 8*, 443–478.

Ingram, R. E. (1990). Self-focused attention in clinical disorders: Review and a conceptual model. *Psychological Bulletin, 107*, 156–176.

Ingram, R. E. (1991). Tilting at windmills: A Response to Pyszczynski, Greenberg, Hamilton, and Nix. *Psychological Bulletin, 110*, 544–550.

Ingram, R. E., Bailey, K., & Siegle, G. J. (2004). Emotional information processing and disrupted parental bonding: Cognitive specificity and avoidance. *Journal of Cognitive Psychotherapy, 18*, 53–65.

Ingram, R. E., Bernet, C. Z., & McLaughlin, S. C. (1994). Attentional allocation processes in individuals at risk for depression. *Cognitive Therapy and Research, 18*, 317–332.

Ingram, R. E., Cruet, D., Johnson, B., & Wisnicki, K. S. (1988). Self-focused attention, gender, gender role, and vulnerability to negative affect. *Journal of Personality and Social Psychology, 55*, 967–978.

Ingram, R. E., & Hollon, S. D. (1986). Cognitive therapy of depression from an information processing perspective. In R. E. Ingram (Ed.), *Information processing approaches to clinical psychology* (pp. 259–281). San Diego: Academic Press.

Ingram, R. E., Johnson, B. R., Bernet, C. Z., Dombeck, M., & Rowe, M. K. (1992). Cognitive and emotional reactivity in chronically self-focused individuals. *Cognitive Therapy and Research, 16*, 451–472.

Ingram, R. E., & Kendall, P. C. (1986). Cognitive clinical psychology: Implications of an information processing perspective. In R. E. Ingram (Ed.), *Information processing approaches to clinical psychology* (pp. 4–21). Orlando, FL: Academic Press.

Ingram, R. E. (Ed.). (1986). *Information processing approaches to clinical psychology*. Orlando, FL: Academic Press.

Ingram, R. E., & Luxton, D. (2005). Vulnerability-stress models. In B. L. Hankin & J. R. Z. Abela (Eds.), *Development of psychopathology: A vulnerability-stress perspective* (pp. 32–46). New York: Sage.

Ingram, R. E., Miranda, J. E., & Segal, Z. V. (1998). *Cognitive vulnerability to depression*. New York: Guilford Press.

Ingram, R. E., Overbey, T., & Fortier, M. (2001). Individual differences in dysfunctional automatic thinking and parental bonding: Specificity of maternal care. *Personality and Individual Differences, 30*, 401–412.

Ingram, R. E., & Price, J. (2010). Understanding psychopathology the role of vulnerability in understanding psychopathology. In R. E. Ingram & J. Price (Eds.), *Vulnerability to psychopathology: Risk across the lifespan* (pp. 3–17). New York: Guilford Press.

Ingram, R. E., & Ritter, J. (2000). Vulnerability to depression: Cognitive reactivity and parental bonding in high-risk individuals. *Journal of Abnormal Psychology, 109*, 588–596.

Ingram, R. E., & Ritter, J. (2007). Vulnerability to depression: Cognitive reactivity and parental bonding in high-risk individuals. *Journal of Abnormal Psychology, 109,* 588–596.

Ingram, R. E., & Smith, T. W. (1984). Depression and internal versus external focus of attention. *Cognitive Therapy and Research, 8,* 139–152.

Ito, H., Kawashima, R., Awata, S., Ono, S., Sato, K., Goto, R., et al. (1996). Hypoperfusion in the limbic system and prefrontal cortex in depression: SPECT with anatomic standardization technique. *Journal of Nuclear Medicine, 37,* 410.

Jabbi, M., Korf, J., Kema, I. P., Hartman, C., van der Pompe, G., Minderaa, R. B., et al. (2007). Convergent genetic modulation of the endocrine stress response involves polymorphic variations of 5-HTT, COMT and MAOA. *Molecular Psychiatry, 12,* 483–490.

Jacobs, N., Kenis, G., Peeters, F., Derom, C., Vlietinck, R., & van Os, J. (2006). Stress-related negative affectivity and genetically altered serotonin transporter function: Evidence of synergism in shaping risk of depression. *Archives of General Psychiatry, 63,* 989–996.

Jaeger, J., Borod, J. C., & Peselow, E. (1986). Facial expressions of positive and negative emotions in patients with unipolar depression. *Journal of Affective Disorders, 11,* 43–50.

James, W. (1884). What is an emotion? *Mind, 9,* 188–205.

Jarrett, R., Kraft, D., Doyle, J., Foster, B., Eaves, G., & Silver, P. (2001). Preventing recurrent depression using cognitive therapy with and without a continuation phase. *Archives of General Psychiatry, 58,* 381–388.

Jha, A., Krompinger, J., & Baime, M. (2007). Mindfulness training modifies subsystems of attention. *Cognitive Affective and Behavioral Neuroscience, 7,* 109–119.

Johnson, S. L., Winett, C. A., Meyer, B., Greenhouse, W. J., & Miller, I. (1999). Social support and the course of bipolar disorder. *Journal of Abnormal Psychology, 108*(4), 558–566.

Joiner, T., & Coyne, J. (Eds.). (1999). *The interactional nature of depression: Advances in interpersonal approaches.* Washington, DC: American Psychological Association.

Jones, N. A., Field, T., Davalos, M., & Pickens, J. (1997). EEG stability in infants/children of depressed mothers. *Child Psychiatry and Human Development, 28,* 59–70.

Jones, N. A., Field, T., Fox, N. A., Davalos, M., Lundy, B., & Hart, S. (1998). Newborns of mothers with depressive symptoms are physiologically less developed. *Infant Behavior and Development, 21,* 537–541.

Joormann, J., Talbot, L., & Gotlib, I. H. (2007). Biased processing of emotional information in girls at risk for depression. *Journal of Abnormal Psychology, 116,* 135–143.

Jordan, A., & Cole, D. A. (1996). Relation of depressive symptoms to the structure of self-knowledge in childhood. *Journal of Abnormal Psychology, 105,* 530–540.

Kabat-Zinn, J. (1990). *Full catastrophe living: Using the wisdom of your mind to face stress, pain and illness.* New York: Dell.

Kabat-Zinn, J., Lipworth, L., & Burney, R. (1985). The clinical use of mindfulness meditation for the self-regulation of chronic pain. *Journal of Behavioral Medicine, 8*, 163–190.

Kaelber, C. T., Moul, D. E., & Farmer, M. E. (1995). Epidemiology of depression. In E. E. Beckham & W. R. Leber (Eds.), *Handbook of depression* (2nd ed.). New York: Guilford Press.

Kahneman, D. (1973). *Attention and effort.* Englewood Cliffs, NJ: Prentice-Hall.

Kalin, N., Shelton, S., Fox, A., Rogers, J., Oakes, T., & Davidson, R. (2008). The serotonin transporter genotype is associated with intermediate brain phenotypes that depend on the context of eliciting stressor. *Molecular Psychiatry, 13*, 1021–1027.

Kaltenthaler, E., Parry, G., Beverley, C., & Ferriter, M. (2008). Computerised cognitive-behavioural therapy for depression: Systematic review. *British Journal of Psychiatry, 193*, 181–184.

Kalueff, A. V., & La Porte, J. L. (2008). *Behavioral models in stress research.* Hauppauge, NY: Nova Biomedical Books.

Kandel, D. B., & Davies, M. (1982). Epidemiology of depressive mood in adolescents: An empirical study. *Archives of General Psychiatry, 39*, 1205–1212.

Kandel, E., Mednick, S. A., Kirkegaard-Sorensen, L., Hutchings, B., Knop, J., Rosenberg, R., et al. (1988). IQ as a protective factor for subjects at high risk for antisocial behavior. *Journal of Consulting and Clinical Psychology, 56*, 224–226.

Kanfer, F. H., & Hagerman, S. M. (1985). Behavior therapy and the information processing paradigm. In S. Reiss & R. R. Bootzin (Eds.), *Theoretical issues in behavior therapy* (pp. 3–33). New York: Academic Press.

Kapczinski, F., Curran, H. V., Gray, J., & Lader, M. (1994). Flumazentil has an anxiolytic effect in simulated stress. *Psychopharmacology, 114*, 187–189.

Kasl, S. V. (1983). Pursuing the link between stressful life experiences and disease: A time for reappraisal. In C. L. Cooper (Ed.), *Stress research* (pp. 13–26). New York: Wiley.

Katz, M. M., Secunda, S. K., Hirschfeld, R. M., & Koslow, S. H. (1979). NIMH Clinical Research Branch Collaborative Program on the Psychobiology of Depression. *Archives of General Psychiatry, 36*, 765–771.

Kayser, J., Bruder, G., Tenke, C., Stewart, J., & Quitkin, F. (2000). Event-related potentials (ERPs) to hemifield presentations of emotional stimuli: Differences between depressed patients and healthy adults in P3 amplitude and asymmetry. *International Journal of Psychophysiology, 36*, 211–236.

Kazdin, A. E. (1992). *Research design in clinical psychology.* Boston: Allyn & Bacon.

Kazdin, A. E. (2003). *Methodological issues and strategies in clinical research* (3rd ed.). Washington, DC: American Psychological Association.

Keedwell, P. A., Andrew, C., Williams, S. C. R., Brammer, M. J., & Phillips, M. L. (2005). A double dissociation of ventromedial prefrontal cortical responses to sad and happy stimuli in depressed and healthy individuals. *Biological Psychiatry, 58*, 495–503.

Keightley, M., Seminowicz, D., Bagby, R., Costa, P., Fossati, P., & Mayberg, H. (2003). Personality influences limbic–cortical interactions during sad mood induction. *NeuroImage, 20*, 2031–2039.

Keller, M. B. (1985). Chronic and recurrent affective disorders: Incidence, course, and influencing factors. In D. Kemali & G. Recagni (Eds.), *Chronic treatments in neuropsychiatry* (pp. 7–18). New York: Raven Press.

Keller, M. B., Lavori, P. W., Endicott, J., Coryell, W., & Klerman, G. (1983). "Double depression": Two-year follow-up. *American Journal of Psychiatry, 140*, 689–694.

Keller, M. B., Shapiro, R. W., Lavori, P. W., & Wolfe, N. (1982). Relapse in RDC major depressive disorders: Analysis with the life table. *Archives of General Psychiatry, 39*, 911–915.

Kendall, P. C., & Butcher, J. N. (Eds.). (1982). *Handbook of research methods in clinical psychology*. New York: Wiley.

Kendall, P. C., Hollon, S. D., Beck, A. T., Hammen, C. L., & Ingram, R. E. (1987). Issues and recommendations regarding use of the Beck Depression Inventory. *Cognitive Therapy and Research, 11*, 289–299.

Kendall-Tackett, K. A., Williams, L. M., & Finkelhor, D. (1993). Impact of sexual abuse on children: A review and synthesis of recent empirical studies. *Psychological Bulletin, 113*, 164–180.

Kendell, R. E. (1970). Relationship between aggression and depression: Epidemiological implications of a hypothesis. *Archives of General Psychiatry, 22*, 308–318.

Kendler, K. S., Gardner, C., & Prescott, C. (2002). Toward a comprehensive developmental model for major depression in women. *American Journal of Psychiatry, 159*, 1133.

Kendler, K. S., Gatz, M., Gardner, C., & Pedersen, N. (2006). Personality and major depression: A Swedish longitudinal, population-based twin study. *Archives of General Psychiatry, 63*, 1113.

Kendler, K. S., Gatz, M., Gardner, C. O., & Pedersen, N. L. (2005). Age at onset and familial risk for major depression in a Swedish national twin sample. *Psychological Medicine, 35*, 1573–1579.

Kendler, K. S., Kuhn, J. W., Vittum, J., Prescott, C. A., & Riley B. (2005). The interaction of stressful life events and a serotonin transporter polymorphism in the prediction of episodes of major depression: A replication. *Archives of General Psychiatry, 62*, 529–535.

Kendler, K. S., Neale, M. C., Kessler, R. C., Heath, A. C., Kuhn, J. W., & Riley, R. (1992). Familial influences on the clinical characteristics of major depression: A twin study. *Acta Psychiatrica Scandinavica, 86*, 371–378.

Kessler, D., Lewis, G., Kaur, S., Wiles, N., King, M., Weich, S., et al. (2009).

Therapist-delivered Internet psychotherapy for depression in primary care: A randomised controlled trial. *The Lancet, 374,* 628–634.

Kessler, K., & Mayberg, H. (2007). Targeting abnormal neural circuits in mood and anxiety disorders: From the laboratory to the clinic. *Nature Neuroscience, 10,* 1116–1124.

Kessler, R. C. (2002). The categorical versus dimensional assessment controversy in the sociology of mental illness. *Journal of Health and Social Behavior, 43,* 171–188.

Kessler, R. C., Akiskal, H., Ames, M., Birnbaum, H., Greenberg, P., Hirschfeld, R. M., et al. (2006). Prevalence and effects of mood disorders on work performance in a nationally representative sample of U.S. Workers. *The American Journal of Psychiatry, 163,* 1561–1568.

Kessler, R. C., Berglund, P., Demler, O., Jin, R., Koretz, D., Merikangas, K., et al. (2003). The epidemiology of major depressive disorder: Results from the National Comorbidity Survey Replication (NCS-R). *Journal of the American Medical Association, 89,* 3095–3105.

Kessler, R. C., Birnbaum, H., Bromet, E., Hwang, I., Sampson, N., & Shahly, V. (2010). Age differences in major depression: Results from the National Comorbidity Survey Replication (NCS-R). *Psychological Medicine, 40,* 225–237.

Kessler, R. C., McGonagle, K. A., Swartz, M., Blazer, D. G., & Nelson, C. B. (1993). Sex and depression in the National Comorbidity Survey: I. Lifetime prevalence, chronicity and recurrence. *Journal of Affective Disorders, 29,* 85–96.

Kessler, R. C., McGonagle, K. A., Zhao, S., Nelson, C. B., Hughes, M., Eshleman, S., et al. (1994). Lifetime and 12-month prevalence of results from the National Comorbidity Survey. *Archives of General Psychiatry, 51,* 8–19.

Kessler, R. C., & Wang, P. S. (2009). Epidemiology of depression. In I. H. Gotlib & C. L. Hammen (Eds.), *Handbook of depression* (2nd ed., pp. 5–22). New York: Guilford Press.

Kety, S. S., Rosenthal, D., Wender, P. H., & Schulsinger, F. (1968). The types and prevalence of mental illness in the biological and adoptive families of adopted schizophrenics. In D. Rosenthal & S. S. Kety (Eds.), *Transmission of schizophrenia* (pp. 345–362). Oxford, UK: Pergamon Press.

Kim, J., & Diamond, D. (2002). The stressed hippocampus, synaptic plasticity and lost memories. *Nature Reviews Neuroscience, 3,* 453–462.

Kim, S. H., & Hamann, S. (2007). Neural correlates of positive and negative emotion regulation. *Journal of Cognitive Neuroscience, 19,* 776–798.

Klein, D., Depue, R. A., & Krauss, S. P. (1986). Social adjustment in the offspring of parents with bipolar affective disorder. *Journal of Psychopathology and Behavioral Assessment, 8,* 355–366.

Klein, D. N. (2008). Classification of depressive disorders in the DSM-V: Proposal for a two-dimension system. *Journal of Abnormal Psychology, 117,* 552–560.

Klerman, G. L., Lavori, P. W., Rice, J., Reich, T., Endicott, J., Andreasen, N.

C., et al. (1985). Birth-cohort trends in rates of major depressive disorder among relatives of patients with affective disorder. *Archives of General Psychiatry, 42*, 689–693.

Klerman, G. L., Weissman, M. M., Rounsaville, B. J., & Chevron, E. S. (1984). *Interpersonal psychotherapy of depression.* New York: Basic Books.

Knowles, J. B., & Maclean, A. W. (1990). Age-related changes in sleep depressed and healthy subjects: A meta-analysis. *Neuropsychopharmacology, 3*, 251–259.

Kocsis, J. H., Thase, M. E., Trivedi, M. H., Shelton, R. C., Kornstein, S. G., Nemeroff, C. B., et al. (2007). Prevention of recurrent episodes of depression with venlafaxine ER in a 1-year maintenance phase from the PREVENT Study. *Journal of Clinical Psychiatry, 68*, 1014–1023.

Koenigs, M., & Grafman, J. (2009). The functional neuroanatomy of depression: Distinct roles for ventromedial and dorsolateral prefrontal cortex. *Behavioural Brain Research, 201*, 239–243.

Koenigs, M., Huey, E. D., Calamia, M., Raymont, V., Tranel, D., & Grafman, J. (2008). Distinct regions of prefrontal cortex mediate resistance and vulnerability to depression. *Journal of Neuroscience, 28*, 12341–12348.

Kronenberg, G., van Elst, L. T., Regen, F., Deuschle, M., Heuser, I., & Colla, M. (2009). Reduced amygdala volume in newly admitted psychiatric inpatients with unipolar major depression. *Biological Psychiatry, 65*, 735.

Kumano, H., Ida, I., Oshima, A., Takahashi, K., Yuuki, N., Amanuma, M., et al. (2007). Brain metabolic changes associated with predispotion to onset of major depressive disorder and adjustment disorder in cancer patients: A preliminary PET study. *Journal of Psychiatric Research, 41*, 591–599.

Kumar, P., Waiter, G., Ahearn, T., Milders, M., Reid, I., & Steele, J. (2008). Abnormal temporal difference reward-learning signals in major depression. *Brain, 131*, 2084.

Kuyken, W., & Brewin, C. R. (1995). Autobiographical memory functioning in depression and reports of early abuse. *Journal of Abnormal Psychology, 104*, 585–591.

Kuyken, W., Byford, S., Taylor, R. S., Watkins, E., Holden, E., White, K., et al. (2008). Mindfulness-based cognitive therapy to prevent relapse in recurrent depression. *Journal of Consulting and Clinical Psychology, 76*, 966–978.

Lacasse, J., & Leo, J. (2005). Serotonin and depression: A disconnect between the advertisements and the scientific literature. *PLoS Medicine, 2*, 1211.

Lane, R. D., & Nadel, L. (Eds.). (2000). *Cognitive neuroscience of emotion.* New York: Oxford University Press.

Lane, R. D., Nadel, L., Allen, J. J. B., & Kaszniak, A. W. (2000). The study of emotion from the perspective of cognitive neuroscience. In R. Lane, L. Nadel, G. Ahern, J. Allen, A. W. Kaszniak, S. Rapcsak, et al. (Eds.), *Cognitive neuroscience of emotion* (pp. 3–11). New York: Oxford University Press.

Lane, R., Reiman, E., Bradley, M., Lang, P., Ahern, G., Davidson, R., et al. (1997). Neuroanatomical correlates of pleasant and unpleasant emotion. *Neuropsychologia, 35*, 1437–1444.

Lang, P. (1984). Cognition in emotion: Concept and action. In E. Izard, J. Kagan, & R. Zajonc (Eds.), *Emotions, cognition and behavior* (pp. 192–226). Cambridge: Cambridge University Press.

Lang, P., Bradley, M., & Cuthbert, B. (1999). International affective picture system (IAPS): Instruction manual and affective ratings. *The Center for Research in Psychophysiology, University of Florida*.

Lange, C., & James, W. (1922). *The emotions*. New York: Williams and Wilkins Company.

Lau, J., & Eley, T. (2008). Disentangling gene-environment correlations and interactions on adolescent depressive symptoms. *Journal of Child Psychology and Psychiatry, 49*, 142–150.

Lau, M. A., Bishop, S. R., Segal, Z. V., Buis, T., Anderson, N. D., Carlson, L., et al. (2006). The Toronto Mindfulness Scale: Development and validation. *Journal of Clinical Psychology, 62*, 1445–1467.

Lazarus, R. (1984). On the primacy of cognition. *American Psychologist, 39*, 124–129.

Lazarus, R. S. (1982). Thoughts on the relations between emotion and cognition. *American Psychologist, 37*, 1019–1024.

Lazarus, R. S. (1990). Theory-based stress management. *Psychological Inquiry, 1*, 3–13.

Lazarus, R. S., & Folkman, S. (1984). *Stress, appraisal, and coping*. New York: Springer.

LeDoux, J. (1998). *The emotional brain: The mysterious underpinnings of emotional life*. New York: Touchstone Books.

LeDoux, J. (2000). Cognitive-emotional interactions: Listen to the brain. In R. D. Lane & L. Nadel (Eds.), *Cognitive neuroscience of emotion. Series in affective science* (pp. 129–155). New York: Oxford University Press.

Lehmann, H. J. (1959). Psychiatric concepts of depression: Nomenclature and classification. *Canadian Psychiatric Association Journal Supplement, 4*, 1–12.

Lesch, K. P., Bengel, D., Heils, A., Sabol, S. Z., Greenberg, B. D., Petri, S., et al. (1996). Association of anxiety-related traits with a polymorphism in the serotonin transporter gene regulatory region. *Science, 274*, 1527–1531.

Leussis, M., & Andersen, S. (2008). Is adolescence a sensitive period for depression?: Behavioral and neuroanatomical findings from a social stress model. *Synapse: New York, 62*, 22.

Levin, R. L., Heller, W., Mohanty, A., Herrington, J. D., & Miller, G. A. (2007). Cognitive deficits in depression and functional specificity of regional brain activity. *Cognitive Therapy and Research, 31*, 211–233.

Lewinsohn, P. M. (1985). A behavioral approach to depression. In J. C. Coyne (Ed.), *Essential papers in depression*. New York: New York University Press.

Lewinsohn, P. M., & Hoberman, H. M. (1982). Depression. In A. S. Bellack, M. Hersen, & A. E. Kazdin (Eds.), *International handbook of behavior modification and therapy* (pp. 397–429). New York: Plenum Press.

Lewinsohn, P. M., Hops, H., Roberts, R. E., Seeley, J. R., & Andrews, J. A. (1993). Adolescent psychopathology: I. Prevalence and incidence of depression and other DSM-III-R disorders in high school students. *Journal of Abnormal Psychology, 102*, 133–144.

Lewinsohn, P. M., Steinmetz, L., Larson, D. W., & Franklin, J. (1981). Depression-related cognitions: Antecedent or consequence? *Journal of Abnormal Psychology, 90*, 213–219.

Lin, E. H., Von Korff, M., Katon, W., Bush, T., Simon, G. E., Walker, E., et al. (1995). The role of the primary care physician in patients' adherence to antidepressant therapy. *Medical Care, 33*, 67–74.

Linden, D. (2005). The p300: Where in the brain is it produced and what does it tell us? *The Neuroscientist, 11*, 563–576.

Linehan, M. M. (1993). *Cognitive-behavioral treatment of borderline personality disorder*. New York: Guilford Press.

Liotti, M., & Mayberg, H. S. (2001). The role of functional neuroimaging in the neuropsychology of depression. *Journal of Clinical and Experimental Neuropsychology, 23*, 121–136.

Liotti, M., Mayberg, H., McGinnis, S., Brannanm, S., & Jerabek, P. (2002). Unmasking disease-specific cerebral blood flow abnormalities: Mood challenge in patients with remitted unipolar depression. *American Journal of Psychiatry, 159*, 1830–1840.

Luck, S. J., Heinze, H. J., Mangun, G. R., & Hillyard, S. A. (1990). Visual event-related potentials in index focused attention with bilateral stimulus arrays: Functional dissociation of P1 and N1 components. *Electroencephalography and Clinical Neurophysiology, 75*, 528–542.

Luthar, S. S., & Zigler, E. (1991). Vulnerability and competence: A review of research on resilience in childhood. *American Journal of Orthopsychiatry, 61*, 6–22.

Lutz, A., Slagter, H. A., Dunne, J. D., & Davidson, R. J. (2008). Cognitive-emotional interactions: Attention regulation and monitoring in meditation. *Trends in Cognitive Sciences, 12*, 163–169.

Lutz, A., Slagter, H. A., Rawlings, N. B., Francis, A. D., Greischar, L. L., & Davidson, R. J. (2009). Mental training enhances attentional stability: Neural and behavioral evidence. *Journal of Neuroscience, 29*, 13418–13427.

Ma, N., Li, L. J., Shu, N., Liu, J., Gong, G. L., He, Z., et al. (2007). White-matter abnormalities in first-episode, treatment-naive young adults with major depressive disorder. *American Journal of Psychiatry, 164*, 823–826.

Ma, S. H., & Teasdale, J. D. (2004). Mindfulness-based cognitive therapy for depression: Replication and exploration of differential relapse prevention effects. *Journal of Consulting and Clinical Psychology, 72*, 31–40.

Mackinnon, A., Griffiths, K. M., & Christensen, H. (2008). Comparative randomised trial of online cognitive-behavioural therapy and an information website for depression: 12-month outcomes. *British Journal of Psychiatry, 192*, 130–134.

MacQueen, G. M., Campbell, S., McEwen, B., Macdonald, K., & Young, T.

(2003). Course of illness, hippocampal function and volume in major depression. *Biological Psychiatry*, *53*, 87.

Mahoney, M. J. (1977). Reflections on the cognitive-learning trend in psychotherapy. *American Psychologist*, *32*, 5–13.

Mahoney, M. J. (1990). *Human change processes*. New York: Basic Books.

Mak, A. K. Y., Hu, Z. G., Zhang, J. X., Xiao, Z. W., & Lee, T. M. C. (2009). Neural correlates of regulation of positive and negative emotions: An fMRI study. *Neuroscience Letters*, *457*(2), 101–106.

Mannie, Z. N., Norbury, R., Murphy, S. E., Inkster, B., Harmer, C. J., & Cowen, P. J. (2008). Affective modulation of anterior cingulate cortex in young people at increased familial risk of depression. *British Journal of Psychiatry*, *192*, 356–361.

Marsella, A. J., Sartorius, M., Jablensky, A., & Fenton, F. R. (1985). Cross-cultural studies of depressive disorders: An overview. In A. Kleinman & B. Good (Eds.), *Culture and depression: Studies in the anthropology and cross-cultural psychiatry of affect and disorder* (pp. 299–324). Berkeley and Los Angeles: University of California Press.

Martell, C. R., Addis, M. E., & Jacobson, N. S. (2001). *Depression in context: Strategies for guided action*. New York: Norton.

Martin-Soelch, C. (2009). Is depression associated with dysfunction of the central reward system? *Biochemical Society Transactions*, *37*, 313–317.

Mayberg, H. S., Liotti, M., Brannan, S. K., McGinnis, S., Mahurin, R. K., Jerabek, P. A., et al. (1999). Reciprocal limbic–cortical function and negative mood: Converging PET findings in depression and normal sadness. *American Journal of Psychiatry*, *156*, 675–682.

Mayberg, H. S., Lozano, A. M., Voon, V., McNeely, H. E., Seminowicz, D., Hamani, C., et al. (2005). Deep brain stimulation for treatment-resistant depression. *Neuron*, *45*, 651–660.

Mayberg, H. S., Robinson, R., Wong, D., Parikh, R., Bolduc, P., Starkstein, S., et al. (1988). PET imaging of cortical S2 serotonin receptors after stroke: Lateralized changes and relationship to depression. *American Journal of Psychiatry*, *145*, 937–943.

McCabe, C., Cowen, P., & Harmer, C. (2009). Neural representation of reward in recovered depressed patients. *Psychopharmacology*, *205*, 667–677.

McCabe, S., Gotlib, H., & Martin, R. (2000). Cognitive vulnerability for depression: Deployment of attention as a function of history of depression and current mood state. *Cognitive Therapy and Research*, *24*, 427–444.

McCranie, E. W., & Bass, J. D. (1984). Childhood family antecedents of dependency and self-criticism: Implications for depression. *Journal of Abnormal Psychology*, *93*, 3–8.

McEwen, B. S., & Magarinos, A. M. (2001). Stress and hippocampal plasticity: Implications for the pathophysiology of affective disorders. *Human Psychopharmacology: Clinical and Experimental*, *16*, 7–19.

McFarlane, A. H., Norman, G. R., Streiner, D. L., Roy, R., & Scott, D. J. (1980). A longitudinal study of the influence of the psychosocial environment on health status: A preliminary report. *Journal of Health and Social Behavior,* *21,* 124–133.

McKim, R. D. (2008). Rumination as a mediator of the effects of mindfulness: Mindfulness-based stress reduction (MBSR) with a heterogeneous community sample experiencing anxiety, depression, and/or chronic pain. *Dissertation Abstracts International: Section B: The Sciences and Engineering,* *68* (11-B).

Mednick, S. A., & Schulsinger, F. (1968). Some premorbid characteristics related to breakdown in children of schizophrenic mothers. *Journal of Psychiatric Research,* *6,* 267–291.

Meehl, P. E. (1962). Schizotaxia, schizotypy, schizophrenia. *American Psychologist,* *17,* 827–838.

Meltzer, C. C., Smith, G., DeKosky, S. T., Pollock, B. G., Mathis, C. A., Moore, R. Y., et al. (1998). Serotonin in aging, late-life depression, and Alzheimer's disease: The emerging role of functional imaging. *Neuropsychopharmacology,* *18,* 407–430.

Mervaala, E., Fohr, J., Kononen, M., Valkonen-Korhonen, M., Vainio, P., Partanen, K., et al. (2000). Quantitative MRI of the hippocampus and amygdala in severe depression. *Psychological Medicine,* *30,* 117–125.

Meyer, J., Kapur, S., Houle, S., DaSilva, J., Owczarek, B., Brown, G., et al. (1999). Prefrontal cortex 5-HT2 receptors in depression: An [18F] setoperone PET imaging study. *American Journal of Psychiatry,* *156,* 1029–1034.

Meyer, J., McMain, S., Kennedy, S., Korman, L., Brown, G., DaSilva, J., et al. (2003). Dysfunctional attitudes and 5-HT2 receptors during depression and self-harm. *American Journal of Psychiatry,* *160,* 90–99.

Miller, E., & Cohen, J. (2001). An integrative theory of prefrontal cortex function. *Annual Review of Neuroscience,* *24,* 167–202.

Millon, T. (1969). *Modern psychopathology.* Philadelphia: Saunders.

Miranda, J., Gross, J., Persons, J., & Hahn, J. (1998). Mood matters: Negative mood induction activates dysfunctional attitudes in women vulnerable to depression. *Cognitive Therapy and Research,* *22,* 363–376.

Miranda, J., & Persons, J. B. (1988). Dysfunctional attitudes are mood-state dependent. *Journal of Abnormal Psychology,* *97,* 76–79.

Miranda, J., Persons, J. B., & Byers, C. (1990). Endorsement of dysfunctional beliefs depends on current mood state. *Journal of Abnormal Psychology,* *99,* 237–241.

Modell, S., Ising, M., Holsboer, F., & Lauer, C. J. (2002). The Munich vulnerability study on affective disorders: Stability of polysomnographic findings over time. *Biological Psychiatry,* *52,* 430–437.

Modell, S., Ising, M., Holsboer, F., & Lauer, C. J. (2005). The Munich vulnerability study on affective disorders: Premorbid polysomnographic profile of affected high-risk probands. *Biological Psychiatry,* *58,* 694–699.

Monk, C. S., Klein, R. G., Telzer, E. H., Schroth, E. A., Mannuzza, S., Moulton, J. L., et al. (2008). Amygdala and nucleus accumbens activation to emotional facial expressions in children and adolescents at risk for major depression. *American Journal of Psychiatry, 165,* 90–98.

Monroe, S., & Harkness, K. (2005). Life stress, the "Kindling" Hypothesis, and the recurrence of depression: Considerations from a life stress perspective. *Psychological Review, 112,* 417–445.

Monroe, S., & Hadjiyannakis, K. (2002). The social environment and depression: Focusing on severe life stress. In I. H. Gotlib & C. L. Hammen (Eds.), *Handbook of depression* (2nd ed., pp. 314–340). New York: Guilford Press.

Monroe, S. M. (1989). Stress and social support: Assessment issues. In N. Schneiderman, S. M. Weiss, & P. G. Kaufman (Eds.), *Handbook of research in cardiovascular behavioral medicine* (pp. 511–526). New York: Plenum Press.

Monroe, S. M. (2008). Modern approaches to conceptualizing and measuring human life stress. *Annual Review of Clinical Psychology, 4,* 33–52.

Monroe, S. M., Kupfer, D. J., & Frank, E. (1992). Life stress and treatment course of recurrent depression: 1. Response during index episode. *Journal of Consulting and Clinical Psychology, 60,* 718–724.

Monroe, S. M., & Reid, M. W. (2009). Life stress and major depression. *Current Directions in Psychological Science, 18,* 68–72.

Monroe, S. M., & Simons, A. D. (1991). Diathesis–stress theories in the context of life stress research: Implications for the depressive disorders. *Psychological Bulletin, 110,* 406–425.

Monroe, S. M., Slavich, G. M., & Georgiades, K. (2009). In I. H. Gotlib & C. L. Hammen (Eds.), *Handbook of depression* (2nd ed., pp. 340–360). New York: Guilford Press.

Moos, R. H., Fenn, C., Billings, A., & Moos, B. (1989). Assessing life stressors and social resources: Applications to alcoholic patients. *Journal of Substance Abuse, 1,* 135–152.

Moos, R. H., & Moos, B. (1992). *Life Stressors and Social Resources Inventory—Adult form manual.* Palo Alto, CA: Stanford University Medical Center, Center for Health Care Evaluation/Department of Veterans Affairs Medical Center.

Moretti, M. M., Segal, Z. V., McCann, C. D., Shaw, B. F., Vella, D., & Miller, D. T. (1996). Self-referent versus other-referent information processing in mildly depressed, clinically depressed and remitted depressed subjects. *Personality and Social Psychology Bulletin, 22,* 68–80.

Morrison, H. L. (Ed.). (1983). *Children of depressed parents: Risk, identification, and intervention.* New York: Grune & Stratton.

Mrazek, P. J., & Haggerty, R. J. (Eds.). (1994). *Reducing risks for mental disorders: Frontiers for preventive intervention research.* Washington, DC: National Academy Press.

Murray, L., Woolgar, M., Cooper, P., & Hipwell, A. (2001). Cognitive vulnerability to depression in 5-year-old children of depressed mothers. *Journal of Child Psychology and Psychiatry, 42,* 891–899.

Murthy, P., Gangadhar, B. N., Janakiramaiah, N., & Subbakrishna, D. K. (1997). Normalization of P300 amplitude following treatment in dysthymia. *Biological Psychiatry, 42,* 740–743.

Nicholson, I. R., & Neufeld, R. W. J. (1992). A dynamic vulnerability perspective on   stress and schizophrenia. *American Journal of Orthopsychiatry, 62,* 117–130.

Nikendei, C., Dengler, W., Wiedemann, G., & Pauli, P. (2005). Selective processing of pain-related word stimuli in subclinical depression as indicated by event-related brain potentials. *Biological Psychology, 70,* 52–60.

Nolen-Hoeksema, S. (1987). Sex differences in unipolar depression: Evidence and theory. *Psychological Bulletin, 101,* 259–282.

Nolen-Hoeksema, S. (1991). Responses to depression and their effects on the duration of depressive episodes. *Journal of Abnormal Psychology, 100,* 569–582.

Nolen-Hoeksema, S. (2000). The role of rumination in depressive disorders and mixed anxiety/depressive symptoms. *Journal of Abnormal Psychology, 109,* 504–511.

Nolen-Hoeksema, S., & Hilt, L. (2009). Gender differences in depression. In I. H. Gotlib & C. L. Hammen (Eds.), *Handbook of depression* (2nd ed., pp. 368–404). New York: Guilford Press.

Nolen-Hoeksema, S., & Jackson, B. (2001). Mediators of the gender differences in rumination. *Psychology of Women Quarterly, 25,* 37–47.

Northoff, G., & Bermpohl, F. (2004). Cortical midline structure and the self. *Trends in Cognitive Science, 8,* 102–107.

Nurcombe, B. (1992). The evolution and validity of the diagnosis of major depression in childhood and adolescence. In D. Cicchetti & S. L. Toth (Eds.), *Developmental perspectives on depression* (pp. 1–28). Rochester, NY: University of Rochester Press.

Ochsner, K., Ray, R., Cooper, J., Robertson, E., Chopra, S., Gabrieli, J., et al. (2004). For better or for worse: Neural systems supporting the cognitive down- and up-regulation of negative emotion. *Neuroimage, 23,* 483–499.

Ochsner, K. N., Bunge, S., Gross, J., & Gabrieli, J. (2002). Rethinking feelings: An fMRI study of the cognitive regulation of emotion. *Journal of Cognitive Neuroscience, 14,* 1215–1229.

Ochsner, K. N., & Gross, J. J. (2008). Cognitive emotion regulation: Insights from social cognitive and affective neuroscience. *Current Directions in Psychological Science, 17,* 153–158.

Oda, K., Okubo, Y., Ishida, R., Murata, Y., Ohta, K., Matsuda, T., et al. (2003). Regional cerebral blood flow in depressed patients with white matter magnetic resonance hyperintensity. *Biological Psychiatry, 53,* 150–156.

Ohira, H. (1996). Accessibility of negative constructs in depression: An event-related brain potential and reaction time analysis. *Japanese Journal of Experimental Social Psychology, 35,* 304–316.

Öhman, A. (1987). The psychophysiology of emotion: An evolutionary-cognitive perspective. *Advances in Psychophysiology, 2,* 79–127.

Öhman, A. (1999). Distinguishing unconscious from conscious emotional processes: Methodological considerations and theoretical implications. In T. Dalgleish & M. Power (Eds.), *Handbook of cognition and emotion* (pp. 321–352). New York: Wiley.

Öhman, A., Flykt, A., & Lundqvist, D. (2000). Unconscious emotion: Evolutionary perspectives, psychophysiological data and neuropsychological mechanisms. In R. D. Lane & L. Nadel (Eds.), *Cognitive neuroscience of emotion. Series in affective science* (pp. 296–327). New York: Oxford University Press.

Olfson, M., Marcus, S., Druss, B., Elinson, L., Tanielian, T., & Pincus, H. (2002). National trends in the outpatient treatment of depression. *Journal of the American Medical Association, 287,* 203–209.

Oltman, J., & Friedman, S. (1964). Relapses following treatment with antidepressant drugs. *Diseases of the Nervous System, 25,* 699–701.

Ormel, J., Oldehinkel, T., Brilman, E., & Vanden Brink, W. (1993). Outcome of depression and anxiety in primary care: A three-wave 3½-year study of psychopathology and disability. *Archives of General Psychiatry, 50,* 759–766.

Ortner, C. N. M., Kilner, S. J., & Zelazo, P. D. (2007). Mindfulness meditation and reduced emotional interference on a cognitive task. *Motivation and Emotion, 31,* 271–283.

Osgood-Hynes, D., Greist, J., Marks, I., Baer, L., Heneman, S., Wenzel, K., et al. (1998). Self-administered psychotherapy for depression using a telephone-accessed computer system plus booklets: An open US–UK study. *Journal of Clinical Psychiatry, 59,* 358–365.

Owens, M. J., & Nemeroff, C. B. (1994). Role of serotonin in the pathophysiology of depression: Focus of the serotonin transporter. *Clinical Chemistry, 40,* 288–295.

Parker, G. (1979). Parental characteristics in relation to depressive disorders. *British Journal of Psychiatry, 134,* 138–147.

Parker, G. (1983). Parental "affectionless control" as an antecedent to adult depression: A risk factor delineated. *Archives of General Psychiatry, 40,* 956–960.

Parker, G., Tupling, H., & Brown, L. (1979). A parental bonding instrument. *British Journal of Medical Psychology, 52,* 1–10.

Pascual-Leone, A., Rubio, B., Pallardo, F., & Catala, M. (1996). Rapid-rate transcranial magnetic stimulation of left dorsolateral prefrontal cortex in drug-resistant depression. *The Lancet, 348,* 233–237.

Paykel, G., Scott, J., Teasdale, J., Johnson, A., Garland, A., Moore, R., et al. (1999). Prevention of relapse in residual depression by cognitive therapy. *Archives of General Psychiatry, 56,* 829–835.

Pearlin, L. I., & Schooler, C. (1978). The structure of coping. *Journal of Health and Social Behavior, 19,* 2–21.

Peck, J. R., Smith, T. W., Ward, J. R., & Milano, F. (1989). Disability and depression in rheumatoid arthritis. A multitrait-multimethod investigation. *Arthritis and Rheumatism, 29,* 1456–1466.

Perez-Edgar, K., Fox, N. A., Cohn, J. F., & Kovacs, M. (2006). Behavioral and electrophysiological markers of selective attention in children of parents with a history of depression. *Biological Psychiatry, 60*, 1131–1138.

Perlis, M., Giles, D., Buysse, D., Thase, M., Tu, X., & Kupfer, D. (1997). Which depressive symptoms are related to which sleep electroencephalographic variables? *Biological Psychiatry, 42*, 904–913.

Persons, J. B. (1986). The advantages of studying psychological phenomena rather than psychiatric diagnoses. *American Psychologist, 41*, 1252–1260.

Persons, J. B., & Miranda, J. (1992). Cognitive theories of depression: Reconciling negative evidence. *Cognitive Therapy and Research, 16*, 485–502.

Persons, J. B., & Rao, P. A. (1985). Longitudinal study of cognitions, life events and depression in psychiatric inpatients. *Journal of Abnormal Psychology, 94*, 51–63.

Pezawas, L., Meyer-Lindenberg, A., Drabant, E. M., Verchinski, B. A., Munoz, K. E., Kolachana, B. S., et al. (2005). 5-HTTLPR polymorphism impacts human cingulate–amygdala interactions: A genetic susceptibility mechanism for depression. *Nature Neuroscience, 8*, 828–834.

Phan, K., Wager, T., Taylor, S., & Liberzon, I. (2004). Functional neuroimaging studies of human emotions. *CNS Spectrums, 9*, 258–266.

Phares, V. (1996). *Fathers and developmental psychopathology*. New York: Wiley.

Phares, V., & Compas, B. E. (1992). The role of fathers in child and adolescent psychopathology: Make room for daddy. *Psychological Bulletin, 111*, 387–412.

Phares, V., Fields, S., Kamboukos, D., & Lopez, E. (2005). Still looking for Poppa. *American Psychologist, 60*, 735–736.

Phillips, D., & Segal, B. (1969). Sexual status and psychiatric symptoms. *American Sociological Review, 34*, 58–72.

Phillips, M. L., Drevets, W. C., Rauch, S. L., & Lane, R. (2003). Neurobiology of emotion perception II: Implications for major psychiatric disorders. *Biological Psychiatry, 54*, 515–528.

Pierson, A., Ragot, R., VanHooff, J., Partiot, A., Renault, B., & Jouvent, R. (1996). Heterogeneity of information-processing alterations according to dimensions of depression: An event-related potentials study. *Biological Psychiatry, 40*, 98–115.

Pilkonis, P., & Frank, E. (1988). Personality pathology in recurrent depression: Nature, prevalence, and relationship to treatment response. *American Journal of Psychiatry, 145*, 435–441.

Pollock, V., Gabrielli, W., Mednick, S., & Goodwin, D. (1988). EEG identification of subgroups of men at risk for alcoholism? *Psychiatry Research, 26*, 101–114.

Portin, R., Kovala, T., Polo-Kantola, P., Revonsuo, A., Muller, K., & Matikainen, E. (2000). Does P3 reflect attentional or memory performances, or cognition more generally? *Scandinavian Journal of Psychology, 41*, 31–40.

Posner, M. I., & McLeod, P. (1982). Information processing models—In search of elementary operations. In M. R. Rosenzweig & L. W. Porter (Eds.), *Annual review of psychology* (Vol. 33, pp. 1–23). Palo Alto, CA: Annual Reviews.

Post, R. M. (1992). Transduction of psychosocial stress into the neurobiology of recurrent affective disorder. *American Journal of Psychiatry, 149,* 999–1010.

Post, R. M. (2007). Kindling and sensitization as models for affective episode recurrence, cyclicity, and tolerance phenomena. *Neuroscience and Biobehavioral Reviews, 31,* 851–873.

Pribram, K. H. (1986). The cognitive revolution and mind/brain issues. *American Psychologist, 41,* 507–520.

Pritchard, W. (1981). Psychophysiology of P300. *Psychological Bulletin, 89,* 506–540.

Proudfoot, J., Ryden, C., Everitt, B., Shapiro, D. A., Goldberg, D., Mann, A., et al. (2004). Clinical efficacy of computerised cognitive-behavioural therapy for anxiety and depression in primary care: Randomised controlled trial. *British Journal of Psychiatry, 185,* 46–54.

Pryce, C. (2008). Postnatal ontogeny of expression of the corticosteroid receptor genes in mammalian brains: Inter-species and intra-species differences. *Brain Research Reviews, 57,* 596–605.

Pyszczynski, T., & Greenberg, J. (1987). Self-regulatory preseveration and the depressive self-focusing style: A self-awareness theory of reactive depression. *Psychological Bulletin, 102,* 1–17.

Radke-Yarrow, M., Belmont, B., Nottelmann, E., & Bottomly, L. (1990). Young children's self-conceptions: Origins in the natural discourse of depressed and normal mothers and their children. In D. Cicchetti & M. Beeghly (Eds.), *The self in transition* (pp. 345–361). Chicago: University of Chicago Press.

Radloff, L. (1975). Sex differences in depression: The effects of occupation and marital status. *Sex Roles, 1,* 249–265.

Ramel, W., Goldin, P. R., Carmona, P. E., & McQuaid, J. R. (2004). The effects of mindfulness meditation on cognitive processes and affect in patients with past depression. *Cognitive Therapy and Research, 28,* 433–455.

Ramel, W., Goldin, P. R., Eyler, L. T., Brown, G. G., Gotlib, I. H., & McQuaid, J. R. (2007). Amygdala reactivity and mood-congruent memory in individuals at risk for depressive relapse. *Biological Psychiatry, 61,* 231–239.

Rao, U., Dahl, R., Ryan, N., Birmaher, B., Williamson, D., Giles, D., et al. (1996). The relationship between longitudinal clinical course and sleep and cortisol changes in adolescent depression. *Biological Psychiatry, 40,* 474–484.

Rao, U., Poland, R., Lutchmansingh, P., Ott, G., McCracken, J., & Lin, K. (1999). Relationship between ethnicity and sleep patterns in normal controls: Implications for psychopathology and treatment. *Journal of Psychiatric Research, 33,* 419–426.

Ravden, D., & Polich, J. (1998). Habituation of P300 from visual stimuli. *International Journal of Psychophysiology, 30*, 359–365.

Regier, D. A., Boyd, J. H., Burke, J. D., Rae, D. S., Myers, J. K., Kramer, M., et al. (1988). One-month prevalence of mental disorders in the United States: Based on five Epidemiologic Catchment Area sites. *Archives of General Psychiatry, 45*, 977–986.

Revicki, D. A., Whitley, T. W., Gallery, M. E., & Allison, E. J., Jr. (1993). Impact of work environment characteristics on work-related stress and depression in emergency medicine residents: A longitudinal study. *Journal of Community and Applied Social Psychology, 3*, 273–284.

Reynolds, C., & Kupfer, D. (1987). Sleep research in affective illness: State of the art circa 1987. *Sleep, 10*, 199–215.

Ricks, M. (1985). The social transmission of parental: Attachment across generations. In I. Bretherton & E. Waters (Eds.), Growing points in attachment theory and research. *Monographs of the Society for Research in Child Development, 50*(1–2, Serial No. 209), 445–466.

Roberts, J., Gotlib, I., & Kassel, J. (1996). Adult attachment security and symptoms of depression: The mediating roles of dysfunctional attitudes and low self-esteem. *Journal of Personality and Social Psychology, 70*, 310–320.

Roberts, M., & Ilardi, S. (Eds.). (2003). *Handbook of research methods in clinical psychology*. New York: Malden Blackwell Publishing.

Robins, L. N., Helzer, J. E., Croughan, J., & Ratcliff, K. S. (1981). National Institute of Mental Health Diagnostic Interview Schedule: Its history, characteristics, and validity. *Archives of General Psychiatry, 38*, 381–389.

Rolf, J. (1972). The social and academic competence of children vulnerable to schizophrenia and other behavior pathologies. *Journal of Abnormal Psychology, 80*, 225–243.

Rolf, J., & Garmezy, M. (1974). The school performance of children vulnerable to behavior pathology. In D. F. Ricks & M. Roff (Eds.), *Life history research in psychopathology* (pp. 202–234). Minneapolis: University of Minnesota Press.

Romano, J. M., & Turner, J. A. (1985). Chronic pain and depression: Does the evidence support a relationship? *Psychological Bulletin, 97*, 18–34.

Roschke, J., Wagner, P., Mann, K., Fell, J., Grozinger, M., & Frank, C. (1996). Single trial analysis of event related potentials: A comparison between schizophrenics and depressives. *Biological Psychiatry, 40*, 844–852.

Rose, D. T., & Abramson, L. Y. (1992). Developmental predictors of depressive cognitive style: Research and theory. In D. Cicchetti & S. L. Toth (Eds.), *Developmental perspectives on depression* (pp. 323–379). Rochester, NY: University of Rochester Press.

Rose, D. T., Abramson, L. Y., Hodulik, C. J., Halberstadt, L., & Leff, G. (1994). Heterogeneity of cognitive style among depressed inpatients. *Journal of Abnormal Psychology, 103*, 419–429.

Rosenthal, D. (1970). *Genetic theory and abnormal behavior*. New York: McGraw-Hill.

Rosenthal, D., Wender, P. H., Kety, S. S., Schulsinger, F., Welner, J., & Oster-gaard, L. (1968). Schizophrenics' offspring reared in adoptive homes. In D. Rosenthal & S. S. Kety (Eds.), *Transmission of schizophrenia* (pp. 171–193). Oxford, UK: Pergamon.

Rudolph, K., & Conley, C. (2005). The socioemotional costs and benefits of social-evaluative concerns: Do girls care too much? *Journal of Personality, 73,* 115–137.

Rusch, B. D., Abercrombie, H. C., Oakes, T. R., Schaefer, S. M., & Davidson, R. J. (2001). Hippocampal morphometry in depressed patients and control subjects: Relations to anxiety symptoms. *Biological Psychiatry, 50,* 960–964.

Rush, J., Kraemer, H., Sackeim, H., Fava, M., Trivedi, M., & Frank, E., et al. (2006). Report by the ACNP Task Force on response and remission in major depressive disorder. *Neuropsychopharmacology, 31,* 1841–1853.

Rutter, M. (1987). Psychosocial resilience and protective mechanisms. *American Journal of Orthopsychiatry, 57,* 316–331.

Rutter, M. (1988a). Longitudinal data in the study of casual processes: Some uses and some pitfalls. In M. Rutter (Ed.), *Studies of psychosocial risk: The power of longitudinal data* (pp. 1–28). Cambridge, UK: Cambridge University Press.

Rutter, M. (Ed.). (1988b). *Studies of psychosocial risk: The power of longitudinal data.* Cambridge, UK: Cambridge University Press.

Rutter, M. (2009). Understanding and testing risk mechanisms for mental disorders. *Journal of Child Psychology and Psychiatry, 50,* 44–52.

Rutter, M., Maughan, B., Mortimore, P., & Ouston, J. (1979). *Fifteen thousand hours: Secondary schools and their effects on children.* London: Open Books.

Sacco, W. P., & Beck, A. T. (1995). Cognitive theory and therapy. In E. E Beckham & W. R. Leber (Eds.), *Handbook of depression* (2nd ed., pp. 329–351). New York: Guilford Press.

Safran, J. D., & Segal, Z. V. (2009). *Interpersonal process in cognitive therapy.* New York: Basic Books.

Schachter, S. S. J. (1962). Cognitive, social and physiological determinants of emotional state. *Psychological Review, 69,* 379–399.

Schaffer, C. E., Davidson, R. J., & Saron, C. (1983). Frontal and parietal electroencephalogram in depressed and nondepressed subjects. *Biological Psychiatry, 18,* 753–762.

Scher, C. D., Ingram, R. E., & Segal, Z. V. (2005). Cognitive reactivity and vulnerability: Empirical evaluation of construct activation and cognitive diathesis in unipolar depression. *Clinical Psychology Review, 25,* 487–510.

Schildkraut, J. (1965). The catecholamine hypothesis of affective disorders: A review of supporting evidence. *American Journal of Psychiatry, 122,* 509.

Schmidt, P. J., Nieman, L. K., Grover, G. N., Muller, K. L., Merriam, G. R., & Rubinow, D. R. (1991). Lack of effect of induced menses on symptoms in women with premenstrual syndrome. *New England Journal of Medicine*, *324*, 1174–1179.

Sears, R. R., Maccoby, E. E., & Levin, H. (1957). *Patterns of childrearing*. Evanston, IL: Row Peterson.

Segal, Z. V. (1988). Appraisal of the self-schema construct in cognitive models of depression. *Psychological Bulletin*, *103*, 147–162.

Segal, Z. V., & Dobson, K. S. (1992). Cognitive models of depression: Report from a consensus conference. *Psychological Inquiry*, *3*, 225–229.

Segal, Z. V., Gemar, M., & Williams, S. (1999). Differential cognitive response to a mood challenge following successful cognitive therapy or pharmacotherapy for unipolar depression. *Journal of Abnormal Psychology*, *108*, 3–10.

Segal, Z. V., & Ingram, R. E. (1994). Mood priming and construct activation in tests of cognitive vulnerability to unipolar depression. *Clinical Psychology Review*, *14*, 663–695.

Segal, Z. V., Kennedy, S., Gemar, M., Hood, K., Pedersen, R., & Buis, T. (2006). Cognitive reactivity to sad mood provocation and the prediction of depressive relapse. *Archives of General Psychiatry*, *63*, 749–755.

Segal, Z. V., Pearson, J. L., & Thase, M. E. (2003). Challenges in preventing relapse in major depression: Report of a National Institute of Mental Health Workshop on state of the science of relapse prevention in major depression. *Journal of Affective Disorders*, *77*, 97–108.

Segal, Z. V., & Shaw, B. F. (1986). Cognition in depression: A reappraisal of Coyne & Gotlib's critique. *Cognitive Therapy and Research*, *10*, 671–694.

Segal, Z. V., Shaw, B. F., Vella, D. D., & Katz, R. (1992). Cognitive and life stress predictors of relapse in remitted unipolar depressed patients: Test of the congruency hypothesis. *Journal of Abnormal Psychology*, *101*, 26–36.

Segal, Z. V., & Vella, D. D. (1990). Self-schema in major depression: Replication and extension of a priming methodology. *Cognitive Therapy and Research*, *14*, 161–176.

Segal, Z. V., Williams, J. M., & Teasdale, J. D. (2002). *Mindfulness-based cognitive therapy for depression: A new approach to preventing relapse*. New York: Guilford Press.

Segrin, C. (2001). Social skills and negative life events: Testing the deficit stress generation hypothesis. *Current Psychology*, *20*, 19–35.

Seligman, M. E. P. (1975). *Helplessness: On depression, development, and death*. San Francisco: Freeman.

Seligman, M. E. P., Schulman, P., DeRubeis, R. J., & Hollon, S. D. (1999, December 21). The prevention of depression and anxiety. *Prevention and Treatment*, *2*, ArtID 8a.

Seligman, M. E. P., Schulman, P., & Tryon, A. M. (2007). Group prevention of depression and anxiety symptoms. *Behaviour Research and Therapy*, *45*, 1111–1126.

Selye, H. (1936). A syndrome produced by diverse nocuous agents. *Nature*, *138*, 32.

Shankman, S. A., Tenke, C. E., Bruder, G. E., Durbin, C. E., Hayden, E. P., & Klein, D. N. (2005). Low positive emotionality in young children: Association with EEG asymmetry. *Development and Psychopathology*, *17*, 85–98.

Shapiro, S. L., & Carlson, L. E. (2009). *The art and science of mindfulness: Integrating mindfulness into psychology and the helping professions*. Washington, DC: American Psychological Association.

Shea, M. T., Elkin, I., Imber, S., Sotsky, S., Watkins, J., Collins, J., et al. (1992). Course of depressive symptoms over follow up: Findings from the NIMH Treatment of Depression Collaborative Research Program. *Archives of General Psychiatry*, *49*, 782–787.

Shea, M. T., Glass, D., Pilkonis, P., Warkins, J., & Docherty, J. (1987). Frequency and implications of personality disorders in a sample of depressed outpatients. *Journal of Personality Disorders*, *1*, 27–42.

Shea, M. T., Leon, A. C., Mueller, T., & Solomon, D. A. (1996). Does major depression result in lasting personality change? *American Journal of Psychiatry*, *153*, 1404–1410.

Sheline, Y. I., Wang, P. W., Gado, M. H., Csernansky, J. G., & Vannier, M. W. (1996). Hippocampal atrophy in recurrent major depression. *Proceedings of the National Academy of Sciences of the United States of America*, *93*, 3908–3913.

Shelton, R. C., Hollon, S. D., Purdon, S. E., & Loosen, P. T. (1991). Biological and psychological aspects of depression. *Behavior Therapy*, *22*, 201–228.

Sher, K. J., & Trull, T. J. (1996). Methodological issues in psychopathology research. *Annual Review of Psychology*, *47*, 371–400.

Siegel, D. J. (2007). *The mindful brain: Reflection and attunement in the cultivation of well-being*. New York: Norton.

Siegle, G. J., Carter, C. S., & Thase, M. E. (2006). Use of fMRI to predict recovery from unipolar depression with cognitive behavior therapy. *American Journal of Psychiatry*, *163*, 735–738.

Siegle, G. J., & Ingram, R. E. (1997). Modeling individual differences in negative information processing biases. In G. Matthews (Ed.), *Cognitive science perspectives on personality and emotion* (pp. 15–39). New York: Elsevier Science.

Siegle, G. J., Steinhauer, S. R., Thase, M. E., Stenger, V. A., & Carter, C. S. (2002). Can't shake that feeling: Event-related fMRI assessment of sustained amygdala activity in response to emotional information in depressed individuals. *Biological Psychiatry*, *51*, 693–707.

Siegle, G. J., Thompson, W., Carter, C., Steinhauser, S., & Thase, M. (2007). Increased amygdala and decreased dorsolateral prefrontal BOLD responses in unipolar depression: Related and independent features. *Biological Psychiatry*, *61*, 198–209.

Simon, G., Fleck, M., Lucas, R., & Bushnell, D. (2004). Prevalence and predictors of depression treatment in an international primary care study. *The American Journal of Psychiatry, 161*, 1626–1634.

Simons, A., Murphy, G., Levine, J., & Wetzel, R. (1986). Cognitive therapy and pharmacotherapy for depression: Sustained improvement over one year. *Archives of General Psychiatry, 43*, 43–50.

Singer, T., Seymour, B., O'Doherty, J., Kaube, H., Dolan, R. J., & Frith, C. D. (2004). Empathy for pain involves the affective but not sensory components of pain. *Science, 303*, 1157–1162.

Slagter, H., Lutz, A., Greischar, L., Francis, A., Nieuwenhuis, S., Davis, J., et al. (2007). Mental training affects distribution of limited brain resources. *PLoS Biology, 5*, 1228–1235.

Smith, A., Henson, R., Dolan, R., & Rugg, M. (2004). fMRI correlates of the episodic retrieval of emotional contexts. *Neuroimage, 22*, 868–878.

Smith, K. A., Ploghaus, A., Cowen, P. J., McCleery, J. M., Goodwin, G. M., Smith, S., et al. (2002). Cerebellar responses during anticipation of noxious stimuli in subjects recovered from depression: Functional magnetic resonance imaging study. *British Journal of Psychiatry, 181*, 411–415.

Smith, T. W., & Rhodewalt, F. T. (1991). Methodological challenges at the social/clinical interface. In C. R. Snyder & D. R. Forsyth (Eds.), *Handbook of social and clinical psychology: The health perspective* (pp. 739–756). New York: Pergamon Press.

Smith, T. W., Wallston, K. A., & Dwyer, K. A. (1995). On babies and bathwater: Disease impact and negative affectivity in the self-reports of persons with rheumatoid arthritis. *Health Psychology, 14*, 64, 73.

Solomon, A., Haaga, D. A. F., & Arnow, B. A. (2001). Is clinical depression distinct from subthreshold depressive symptoms? A review of the continuity issue in depression research. *Journal of Nervous and Mental Disease, 189*, 498–506.

Solomon, A., Haaga, D., Brody, C., Kirk, L., & Friedman, D. (1998). Priming irrational beliefs in recovered-depressed people. *Journal of Abnormal Psychology, 107*, 440–449.

Solomon, A., Ruscio, J., Seeley, J. R., & Lewinsohn, P. M. (2006). A taxometric investigation of unipolar depression in a large community sample. *Psychological Medicine, 36*, 973–985.

Somerset, W., Newport, D. J., Ragan, K., & Stowe, Z. N. (2007). Depressive disorders in women: From menarche to beyond menopause. In C. L. M. Keys & S. H. Goodman (Eds.), *Women and depression* (pp. 62–88). New York: Cambridge University Press.

Spitzer, R. L., & Endicott, J. (1978). Medical and mental disorder: Proposed definition and criteria. In R. L. Spitzer & D. F. Klein (Eds.), *Critical issues in psychiatric diagnosis* (pp. 773–782). New York: Raven Press.

Stark, K. D., Yancy, M., Simpson, J., & Molnar, J. (2007). *Treating depressed children: Therapist manual for parent component of "ACTION."* Ardmore, PA: Workbook Publishing.

Steiner, M., Dunn, E., & Born, L. (2003). Hormones and mood: From menarche to menopause and beyond. *Journal of Affective Disorders, 74*, 67–83.

Sternberg, S. (1969). The discovery of processing stages: Extensions of Donders method. *Acta Psychologia, 30*, 276–315.

Stewart, R. E., & Chambless, D. L. (2009). Cognitive-behavioral therapy for adult anxiety disorders in clinical practice: A meta-analysis of effectiveness studies. *Journal of Consulting and Clinical Psychology, 77*, 595–606.

Stice, E., Burton, E., Bearman, S. K., & Rohde, P. (2006). Randomized trial of a brief depression prevention program: An elusive search for a psychosocial placebo control condition. *Behaviour Research and Therapy, 45*, 863–876.

Taki, Y., Kinomura, S., Awata, S., Inoue, K., Sato, K., Ito, H., et al. (2005). Male elderly subthreshold depression patients have smaller volume of medial part of prefrontal cortex and precentral gyrus compared with age-matched normal subjects: A voxel-based morphometry. *Journal of Affective Disorders, 88*, 313–320.

Tang, T. Z., DeRubeis, R. J., Hollon, S. D., Amsterdam, J., & Shelton, R. (2007). Sudden gains in cognitive therapy of depression and depression relapse/recurrence. *Journal of Consulting and Clinical Psychology, 75*, 404–408.

Taylor, L., & Ingram, R. E. (1999). Cognitive reactivity and depressotypic information processing in the children of depressed mothers. *Journal of Abnormal Psychology, 108*, 202–210.

Teasdale, J. D. (1983). Negative thinking in depression: Cause, effect, or reciprocal relationship? *Advances in Behaviour Therapy and Research, 5*, 3–25.

Teasdale, J. D. (1988). Cognitive vulnerability to persistent depression. *Cognition and Emotion, 2*, 247–274.

Teasdale, J. D., & Barnard, P. J. (1993). *Affect, cognition, and change.* Hillsdale, NJ: Erlbaum.

Teasdale, J. D., & Dent, J. (1987). Cognitive vulnerability to depression: An investigation of two hypotheses. *British Journal of Clinical Psychology, 26*, 113–126.

Teasdale, J. D., Moore, R. G., Hayhurst, H., Pope, M., Williams, S., & Segal, Z. V. (2002). Metacognitive awareness and prevention of relapse in depression: Empirical evidence. *Journal of Consulting and Clinical Psychology, 70*, 275–287.

Teasdale, J. D., Segal, Z. V., & Williams, J. M. (1995). How does cognitive therapy prevent depressive relapse and why should attentional control (mindfulness) training help? *Behaviour Research and Therapy, 33*, 25–39.

Teasdale, J. D., Segal, Z. V., Williams, J. M. G., Ridgeway, V. A., Soulsby, J. M., et al. (2000). Prevention of relapse/recurrence in major depression by mindfulness-based cognitive therapy. *Journal of Consulting and Clinical Psychology, 68*, 615–623.

ten Doesschate, M. C., Bockting, C. L., Koeter, M. W., & Schene, A. H. (2009). Predictors of nonadherence to continuation and maintenance antidepressant medication in patients with remitted recurrent depression. *Journal of Clinical Psychiatry, 70*, 63–69.

ten Doesschate, M. C., Koeter, M. W., Bockting, C. L., Schene, A. H., & DELTA Study Group. (2010). Health related quality of life in recurrent depression: A comparison with a general population sample. *Journal of Affective Disorders*, *120*, 126–132.

Timbremont, B., & Braet, C. (2004). Cognitive vulnerability in remitted depressed children and adolescents. *Behaviour Research and Therapy*, *42*, 423–43.

Tjurmina, O. A., Armando, I., Saavedra, J. M., Goldstein, D. S., & Murphy, D. L. (2002). Exaggerated adrenomedullary response to immobilization in mice with targeted disruption of the serotonin transporter gene. *Endocrinology*, *143*, 4520–4526.

Tolman, E. C. (1932). *Purposive behavior in animals and man*. New York: Century.

Tomarken, A. J., Dichter, G. S., Garber, J., & Simien, C. (2004). Resting frontal brain activity: Linkages to maternal depression and socio-economic status among adolescents. *Biological Psychology*, *67*, 77–102.

Torta, R., Borio, R., Cicolin, A., Vighetti, S., & Ravizza, L. (1994). S-adenosyl-L-methionine normalizes P300 latency in patients with major depression: A preliminary report. *Current Therapeutic Research: Clinical and Experimental*, *55*, 864–874.

Tracy, J., & Robins, R. (2008). The automaticity of emotion recognition. *Emotion*, *8*, 81–95.

Tremblay, L., Naranjo, C., Graham, S., Herrmann, N., Mayberg, H., Hevenor, S., et al. (2005). Functional neuroanatomical substrates of altered reward processing in major depressive disorder revealed by a dopaminergic probe. *Archives of General Psychiatry*, *62*, 1228.

Trivedi, M. H., Rush, A. J., Gaynes, B. N., Stewart, J. W., Wisniewski, S. R., Warden, B., et al. (2007). Maximizing the adequacy of medication treatment in controlled trials and clinical practice: STAR(*)D measurement-based care. *Neuropsychopharmacology*, *32*, 2479–2489.

Trull, T. J., Widiger, T. A., & Guthrie, P. (1990). Categorical versus dimensional status of borderline personality disorder. *Journal of Abnormal Psychology*, *99*, 40–48.

Tucker, D. (1981). Lateral brain function, emotion, and conceptualization. *Psychological Bulletin*, *89*, 19–46.

Tucker, D., & Williamson, P. (1984). Asymmetric neural control systems in human self-regulation. *Psychological Review*, *91*, 185–215.

Twenge, J., & Nolen-Hoeksema, S. (2002). Age, gender, race, socioeconomic status, and birth cohort difference on the children's depression inventory: A meta-analysis. *Journal of Abnormal Psychology*, *111*, 578–588.

van Eijndhoven, P., van Wingen, G., van Oijen, K., Rijpkema, M., Goraj, B., Verkes, R. J., et al. (2009). Amygdala volume marks the acute state in the early course of depression. *Biological Psychiatry*, *65*, 812–818.

Vasta, R., Haith, M. M., & Miller, S. A. (1992). *Child psychology: The modern science*. New York: Wiley.

Veiel, H. O. F. (1997). A preliminary profile of neuropsychological deficits associated with major depression. *Journal of Clinical and Experimental Neuropsychology, 19,* 587–603.

Videbech, P., & Ravnkilde, B. (2004). Hippocampal volume and depression: A meta-analysis of MRI studies. *American Journal of Psychiatry, 161,* 1957–1966.

von Gunten, A., Fox, N. C., Cipolotti, L., & Ron, M. A. (2000). A volumetric study of hippocampus and amygdala in depressed patients with subjective memory problems. *Journal of Neuropsychiatry and Clinical Neurosciences, 12,* 493–498.

Vythilingam, M., Heim, C., Newport, J., Miller, A., Anderson, E., Bronen, R., et al. (2002). Childhood trauma associated with smaller hippocampal volume in women with major depression. *American Journal of Psychiatry, 159,* 2072.

Wagner, G., Sinsel, E., Sobanski, T., Köhler, S., Marinou, V., Mentzel, H., et al. (2006). Cortical inefficiency in patients with unipolar depression: An event-related fMRI study with the Stroop task. *Biological Psychiatry, 59,* 958–965.

Walker, E., & Hoppes, E. (1984). Longitudinal research in schizophrenia: The high risk method. In S. A. Mednick & M. Harway (Eds.), *Handbook of longitudinal research.* New York: Praeger.

Walsh, B. T., Roose, S. P., Glassman, A. H., Gladis, M., & Sadik, C. (1985). Bulimia and depression. *Psychosomatic Medicine, 47,* 123–131.

Waraich, P., Goldner, E., Somers, J., & Hsu, L. (2004). Prevalence and incidence studies of mood disorders: A systematic review. *Canadian Journal of Psychiatry, 2,* 124–138.

Watkins, E., Moberly, N. J., & Moulds, M. L. (2008). Processing mode causally influences emotional reactivity: Distinct effects of abstract versus concrete construal on emotional response. *Emotion, 8,* 364–378.

Weary, G., Edwards, J. A., & Jacobson, J. A. (1995). Depression research methodologies in the *Journal of Personality and Social Psychology*: A reply. *Journal of Personality and Social Psychology, 68,* 885–891.

Weintraub, S. (1987). Risk factors in schizophrenia: The Stony Brook High-Risk Project. *Schizophrenia Bulletin, 13,* 439–450.

Weissman, A., & Beck, A. T. (1978). *Development and validation of the Dysfunctional Attitude Scale: A preliminary investigation.* Paper presented at the meeting of the American Educational Research Association, Toronto, Canada.

Weissman, M., Bruce, M., Leaf, P., Flirio, L., & Holzer, C. (1991). Affective disorders. In L. Robins & D. Regier (Eds.), *Psychiatric disorders in America* (pp. 89–103). New York: Free Press.

Weissman, M. M., Gershon, E. S., Kidd, K. K., Prusoff, B. A., Leckman, J. F., Warner, V., et al. (1984). Psychiatric disorders in the relatives of probands with affective disorders. *Archives of General Psychiatry, 41,* 13–21.

Weissman, M. M., & Klerman, G. L. (1977). Sex differences and the epidemiology of depression. *Archives of General Psychiatry, 34,* 98–111.

Weissman, M. M., & Klerman, G. L. (1985). Gender and depression. *Trends in Neuroscience*, *8*, 416–420.

Weissman, M. M., Klerman, G. L., Prusoff, B. A., Sholomskas, D., & Padian, N. (1981). Depressed outpatients: Results one year after treatment with drugs and/or interpersonal psychotherapy. *Archives of General Psychiatry*, *38*, 52–55.

Weissman, M. M., Leaf, P. J., Holzer, C. E., Myers, J. K., & Tischler, G. L. (1984). The epidemiology of depression: An update on sex differences in rates. *Journal of Affective Disorders*, *7*, 179–188.

Weissman, M. M., Wickramaratne, P., Nomura, Y., Warner, V., Verdeli, H., Pilowsky, D. J., et al. (2005). Families at high and low risk for depression: A 3-generation study. *Archives of General Psychiatry*, *62*, 29–36.

Wells, K. B., Golding, J. M., & Burnam, M. A. (1988). Psychiatric disorder and limitations in physical functioning in a sample of the Los Angeles general population. *American Journal of Psychiatry*, *145*, 712–717.

Wells, K. B., Stewart, A., Hays, R. D., Burnam, M. A., Rogers, W., Daniels, M., et al. (1989). The functioning and wellbeing of depressed patients: Results from the Medical Outcomes Study. *Journal of the American Medical Association*, *262*, 914–919.

Werner, K., & Gross, J. J. (2010). Emotion regulation and psychopathology: A conceptual framework. In A. Kring & D. Sloan (Eds.), *Emotion regulation and psychopathology* (pp. 13–37). New York: Guilford Press.

Westin, D. (1991). Social cognition and object relations. *Psychological Bulletin*, *109*, 429–455.

Whalen, P., Bush, G., McNally, R., Wilhelm, S., McInerney, S., Jenike, M., et al. (1998). The emotional counting Stroop paradigm: A functional magnetic resonance imaging probe of the anterior cingulate affective division. *Biological Psychiatry*, *44*, 1219–1228.

Wheeler, R., Davidson, R., & Tomarken, A. (1993). Frontal brain asymmetry and emotional reactivity: A biological substrate of affective style. *Psychophysiology*, *30*, 82–89.

Whisman, M., & McGarvey, A. (1995). Attachment, depressotypic cognitions, and dysphoria. *Cognitive Therapy and Research*, *19*, 633–650.

Whisman, M. A., & Kwon, P. (1992). Parental representations, cognitive distortions, and mild depression. *Cognitive Therapy and Research*, *16*, 557–568.

Widiger, T. A., & Samuel, D. (2005). Diagnostic categories or dimensions? A question for the Diagnostic and statistical manual of mental disorders (5th ed.). *Journal of Abnormal Psychology*, *114*, 494–504.

Widom, C. (1977). A methodology for studying noninstitutionalized psychopaths. *Journal of Consulting and Clinical Psychology*, *45*, 674–683.

Williams, J. M., Teasdale, J. D., Segal, Z. V., & Kabat-Zinn, J. (2007). *The mindful way through depression: Freeing yourself from chronic unhappiness*. New York: Guilford Press.

Williams, J. M. G., Watts, F. N., MacLeod, C., & Matthews, A. (1988). *Cognitive psychology and emotional disorders*. Chichester, UK: Wiley.

Winokur, G., & Clayton, P. J. (1967). Family history studies: II. Sex differences and alcoholism in primary affective illness. *British Journal of Psychiatry*, *113*, 973–979.

Wolfensberger, S. P. A., Veltman, D. J., Hoogendijk, W. J. G., De Ruiter, M. B., Boomsma, D. I., & de Geus, E. J. C. (2008). The neural correlates of verbal encoding and retrieval in monozygotic twins at low or high risk for depression and anxiety. *Biological Psychology*, *79*, 80–90.

Worland, J., Janes, C., Anthony, E., McGinnis, M., & Cass, L. (1984). St. Louis Risk Research Project: Comprehensive progress report of experimental studies. In N. Watt, E. J. Anthony, L. Wynne, & J. Rolf (Eds.), *Children at risk for schizophrenia* (pp. 105–147). New York: Cambridge University Press.

Worland, J., Weeks, D. G., Janes, C. L., & Strock, B. D. (1984). Intelligence, classroom behavior, and academic achievement in children at high and low risk for psychopathology: A structural equation analysis. *Journal of Abnormal Child Psychology*, *12*, 437–454.

World Health Organization. (1993). *The ICD-10 classification of mental and behavioral disorders: Diagnostic criteria for research*. Geneva, Switzerland: Author.

Yanai, I., Fujikawa, T., Osada, M., Yamawaki, S., & Touhouda, Y. (1997). Changes in auditory P300 in patients with major depression and silent cerebral infarction. *Journal of Affective Disorders*, *46*, 263–271.

Yatham, L., Liddle, P., & Shiah, I. (2000). Brain serotonin receptors in major depression: A positron emission tomography study. *Archives of General Psychiatry*, *57*, 850–858.

Young, J. F., & Mufson, L. (2003). *Manual for interpersonal psychotherapy-adolescent skills training (IPT-AST)*. Unpublished manual, Columbia University, New York, NY.

Zajonc, R. B. (1980). Feeling and thinking: Preferences need no inferences. *American Psychologist*, *35*, 151–175.

Zajonc, R. (1984). On the primacy of affect. *American Psychologist*, *39*, 117–123.

Zhang, Y. Y., Hauser, U., Conty, C., Emrich, H. M., & Dietrich, D. E. (2007). Familial risk for depression and P3b component as a possible neurocognitive vulnerability marker. *Neuropsychobiology*, *55*, 14–20.

Zubin, J., & Spring, B. (1977). Vulnerability—A new view of schizophrenia. *Journal of Abnormal Psychology*, *86*, 103–126.

Zuroff, D., Koestner, R., & Powers, T. A. (1994). Self-criticism at age 12: A longitudinal study of adjustment. *Cognitive Therapy and Research*, *18*, 367–385.

Index

251